AF731055

LIVING ON GO!!!

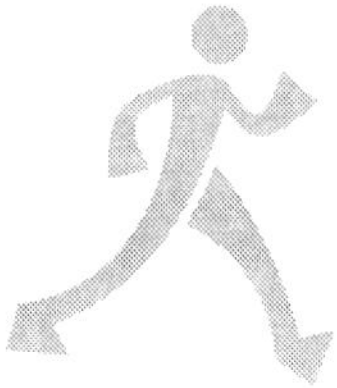

Diane Elms, Hom., D.H.M.H.S., CCII
with Marian den Boer

©2015 Diane Elms

All rights reserved. No part of this publication may be reproduced, distributed, or transmitted in any form or by any means, including photocopying, recording, or other electronic or mechanical methods, without the prior written permission of the publisher, except in the case of brief quotations embodied in critical reviews.

Printed in Canada

ISBN 978-0-9947358-0-5

FIN 10 31 2016

Library and Archives Canada Cataloguing in Publication

Elms, Diane, 1959-, author
Living on go! / Diane Elms & Marian denBoer.

ISBN 978-0-9947358-0-5 (pbk.)

1. Elms, Diane, 1959-. 2. Cancer--Homeopathic treatment--Canada. 3. Homeopathic physicians--Canada--Biography. I. denBoer, Marian, 1952- , author II. Title.

RX66.E45A3 2015 615.5'32092 C2015-903353-5

Contents

Introduction

Life experiences have allowed me to grow, ponder, learn, and relearn as I try to understand who I am. I am fifty-five, and I'm still asking basic questions. Who am I? What am I doing here? What is my purpose? Why do I have to go through so much stuff? I'm thinking these are questions most of us ask.

I believe life is a journey and we never arrive. When we finish one leg of the journey, another begins. We can either embrace the journey or fall victim to it. The choice is ultimately ours. I believe we must embrace the journey and the life lessons that the journey shows us or we miss out. If we do not embrace the journey, *we miss out on life and living!* I believe we only have one chance here on earth. I'm not asking you to believe what I believe, but this is where I am coming from.

I want it all, just call me greedy. I want everything life has to offer. I don't want to miss anything. I have learned that *living* is accepting the journey, walking through the door that opens, even if we have no idea where the door leads. Understand I would not consider myself reckless. I lean conservative in most areas of my life.

About 30 years ago my oldest son Jason was being tested for food allergies. During the session the specialist wrote a note on his pad, tore it off, and handed it to me. I thought this strange. It took me a long time to understand the meaning of his note. He had written, *be content but not satisfied*. Right out of the blue, this doctor who I had never met before stopped doing the allergy testing and he wrote, *be content but not satisfied*. He gave me the note, "This is for you." Then he continued his testing.

I kept that note. Every now and then I would come across the piece of paper, unfold it and reread it. It probably took me 16 years to grasp the meaning of that note. I am glad I finally got it. Yes, life is a never-ending journey.

By the way, I also believe insanity is doing the same thing over and over again and expecting a different result. In other words, get on with the journey.

My journey began nine months previous to March 8, 1959. I am not sure how long my parents knew each other before I was conceived. My mom was seventeen and my father was several years older. They were married sometime between the time I was conceived and the time I was born. I was born Diane Marie McLaughlin at Henderson Hospital in Hamilton Ontario. I didn't know I was born Diane Marie McLaughlin until I was about twelve or thirteen.

I thought I was Diane Marie Beaurivage, until one afternoon at my grandma's apartment. My grandma and I were looking through old photos. Back in those days pictures were all in black and white, square in format, with a white fancy border and stamped with a date at the bottom of the photo. This photo was dated April 1959. It was obvious to me that the picture was of me, I am the oldest grandchild. It had to be me. I was wrapped in a blanket. My mom was holding me in her arms; she was sitting in a lawn chair in the kitchen. The next photo I remember seeing was my mom and this guy all dressed up. The date on the photo was May 1959. Again my mom was holding me in her arms. I was dressed in a christening gown. My grandma told me that was the day I was christened. I asked her who the guy was.

Without missing a beat my grandmother said, "That's your father."

"No it's not."

"That's your father." Grandma was adamant.

I looked at the photo: it didn't look anything like the man I thought of as my father. "It can't be."

"That's your real father." She sifted through the photo box. She brought out another picture of a young man in a uniform, then other photo of this same man standing on a sidewalk somewhere. She produced yet another of this man holding me and my mother standing next to him.

What was going on?

This moment of discovery that things were not what they had seemed became a pivotal moment in my life.

As the story goes, one day my father went out to the store and never came back. I was eighteen months old at the time. My mom was nineteen, on her own with a small child. I give her credit. It couldn't have been easy. She could have given me up for adoption but instead she chose to keep me and endure all that was about to take place in her life and mine.

Time went on and she met Russell Beaurivage. Russell Beaurivage became my father, the only father I knew. Soon after, I had a sister and two brothers. I can see how there was never a need to tell me the truth. My biological father disappeared and never tried to contact me. Nothing was ever mentioned about my biological father until that day with the photos.

My mom had separated from the man whom I called my father just months before that day at my grandmother's. It took my mom a long time to get up the courage to leave. The man I called dad was an alcoholic. He was an abusive, violent alcoholic. But, when he was sober he was awesome. I remember dad illustrated a book for one of my teachers. I had completed a report on the Labrador retriever. He drew an illustration of a lab on the bristol board, that's how it came to be that my teacher asked my dad to illustrate a children's book she had written. He wrote a song. He even taught himself to play the guitar. Yet he never felt good enough about himself to give up the bottle. I understand this now but it wasn't easy to understand as a child, when my dad said he loved me and then did things to me that I knew dads shouldn't do, it was confusing and didn't feel like love.

Finding my dad on the front lawn, passed out drunk as I was leaving to go to school was somewhat embarrassing. Knowing my classmates would be walking past my home to see him didn't make for a comfortable day either.

All these things in life are part of my journey. Getting past the embarrassment and understanding I had no control over what my father did was a huge relief. I know this now but I didn't know it then. I didn't understand it until I started on what so far has been the biggest leg of my journey.

May 1995, I was standing at the trunk of my vehicle lifting out heavy photography equipment. This was my daily routine. As a professional photographer, I wasn't about to let the sun bake my cameras in the trunk of my vehicle where they would undoubtedly accumulate condensation overnight.

On this day something was different. I lifted the equipment out and something felt very *off* in my body. I was due to see my chiropractor the next day, so I dismissed the feeling. By the time I arrived at the chiropractor's office, my arms were tingling, it was difficult for me to lift my arms, and I felt weak. I discussed this with my chiropractor.

I had been seeing a chiropractor regularly for many years. As a child, I had fallen from a three-story apartment building and suffered structural headaches as a result. The chiropractor adjustments helped. On this occasion the chiropractor suggested I come back in a week. This was out of the ordinary: I usually required a once-a-month maintenance appointment. During the week the tingling in my arms extended into my legs and my weakness developed into extreme fatigue. My chiropractor suggested I book an appointment with my family doctor.

After eighteen months involving doctors, specialists, neurologists, psychologists, therapy, a muscle biopsy and pharmaceuticals, I was told there was nothing the medical profession could do for me. During this eighteen month period I had gone from a normal physically active life to barely being able to walk and many days not having the energy to lift my legs or arms.

The worst was not having answers. Having an understanding of what was going on was something I could handle emotionally, physically and mentally. Being told there were no answers—"we have no idea what is going on"—was hard on me. I am an action person. Give me a goal, give me a task and I will complete it. I am a practical visionary, someone who gets an idea and then figures out how to achieve it. This time I had no idea what I was dealing with, no direction, no goal to achieve, and no concept of what to do.

Depression crept into my life, into my mind, and into my body. "Depression" was formerly not even in my vocabulary. This state was totally foreign to me. On the outside I still looked like me but on the inside I didn't know who I was. I no longer had control over my body: it wouldn't do what I wanted it to do. There were days when I no longer had control over my mind.

My children had no idea what was going on. To them I looked the same on the outside but they wondered why I couldn't ride my bike with them. Why I could no longer play ball, run, walk, take them to their events. I can remember one event so clearly. My son Jeff was playing hockey. I brought a blanket to wrap around me while sitting in the arena watching him play. At this point in my journey I could barely lift my legs to walk. It took me quite some time to walk to my seat. My toes dragged with each step and a normal thirty second walk took a lot longer. But getting there wasn't the major challenge that day; the challenge would be leaving.

The game was finished; Jeff had changed into his street clothes, had hockey bag in hand and was ready to leave. I stood up, took a couple of slow steps and that was it. I could not muster the energy to continue to lift my legs. I remember looking at my son and my husband. I truly didn't know what hurt the most, the feeling of sheer panic at not being able to lift my legs, or the looks on their faces. I don't think I could ever adequately describe their looks. Tears streamed down my face. I couldn't move. My husband wanted to pick me up and carry me to our vehicle. I refused. I felt bad enough—I didn't need to draw attention to myself and that's what would have happened if he had carried me out of the arena. They finally convinced me that, with one on either side of me, they could lift me up from my elbows enough that no one would really be able to see what they were doing. My painful muscles had become very rigid and tight, so my husband and son could easily lift me. With very little effort on my part we proceeded out to the truck and home.

Since this physical challenge became my life during those eighteen months a big armchair in our living room overlooking our beautiful front yard became my daily retreat. I could sit in that chair and feel connected to the outside. Our home sat on a hill, surrounded by huge trees, flowering bushes and perennials. You can see why I chose that spot in my time of helplessness.

As a self-employed business owner with three children involved in various activities, I never had time to read. Now, I had plenty of time. So, I started to read the Bible. I had read it before, but one can read the Bible many times and still not get it.

From a very young age I was attracted to church. My extended family and parents did not attend church, but for some reason I was drawn to it. I attended Sunday school at whatever church happened to be in the area of our home. We moved every couple of years so I attended several schools and several churches. I always enjoyed Vacation Bible Schools and I even sang in a choir. When my children were small, I attended church and the children attended Sunday school on a regular basis.

While I was incapacitated, I also began to journal. This was new to me. If you have never kept a journal, I highly recommend it.

During this year and a half, I began to pray or dialogue with God. I call it dialoguing because it isn't what I had perceived as prayer. Prayer had always seemed rigid, conformed, and routine. That was not what I was doing. Sometimes I screamed, most times I cried, sometimes I listened and one time I even asked God to forgive all those people in my life that didn't do what I told them to do. How's that for a prayer? How do I know I actually said that? I read it in my journal. I'm glad to say I've moved along from that place on this journey of mine.

The rest of what is written in this book could be somewhat unbelievable to many. Believe me, in the beginning, it was hard for me to believe what I was living. All that is written is a personal account of actual events in my life. In some cases I have changed people's names but in most cases I have not. The majority of the events involve individuals who can verify the facts.

These events changed my life. These events make me want to say that religion should be outlawed. You might think that is a strange comment coming from someone who is now an ordained minister, but I have observed that many four-walled churches misuse their position or the trust people give them for their own ego or denominational power trip. The word religion is the issue. Religion implies rules and regulations, a follow-me-attitude when it should be a follow-Jesus-attitude. Don't get me wrong, churches, like any other organization need guidelines in order to run safely but that is not what I am talking about. I understand that churches like any other organization are run by humans and humans make mistakes, but in my opinion a church should be different from any other organization.

I truly believe most people want to believe in something bigger then themselves but have a hard time giving up their power, or what they perceive to be their own power to an "unknown" entity. Most people want to be in control and are not about to submit to someone else. Pride and the need to control go hand in hand.

My relationship with God didn't begin until I had the first of many encounters, or as I like to think of them, adventures directed from above—adventures on my journey of life. A relationship is a two-way participatory endeavour. This endeavour is very different from the routine of going to church, sitting in your seat, listening for an hour then going home to do the same thing next Sunday.

I am certain the Holy Spirit had been trying to get my attention for some time, but the first scripture I ever heard from the Lord/Holy Spirit was "John 10:10" I actually heard an audible voice. It freaked me out. I was sitting in my big armchair in the living room; no one else was home at the time. The voice completely caught me off guard. Was I hearing things? I heard it again. I looked to the right and I looked to the left, no one in sight. I was getting scared, what was going on? I heard it one more time, "John 10:10."

I looked up John 10:10 in the Amplified Bible: *The thief comes only in order to steal and kill and destroy. I came that they may have and enjoy life, and have it in abundance.*

"What does that mean?"

I looked up at the ceiling, "Okay God, if you are trying to get my attention you are going to have to do something big so I know it's you." As stated, I was sitting in my big armchair in the living room looking out at the flower garden. A purple hydrangea bush stood directly outside the window. When I asked God to show himself, one of those big purple hydrangea pods on the bush moved—not a little bit but deliberately back and forth in a manner that could not be denied. I thought my mind was going crazy. I am sure I looked like a cartoon character on TV, as I rubbed my eyes in disbelief. Quite frankly, I didn't believe what I was seeing.

It happened again, only this time a different flower on the same bush moved. I quickly looked around to see if the wind was blowing. No wind anywhere. Not a single leaf stirred on this bush or any of the trees or bushes in the front yard. My mind and my heart raced.

Then again, same bush, different flower, while every leaf and every other flower stood as still as still could be. I raised my eyes upward again and asked sheepishly, "Lord is that you?" Every hydrangea pod on that bush shook. I cried and I cried and I cried. I was scared, I was physically shaking. I didn't know what to do and most certainly didn't know who to talk to about this. Who would believe me? I was having a hard time believing it myself.

I kept that bit of information to myself for many, many years before I had the courage and conviction to stand firm in what I had experienced.

Little did I realize this would be the first of many God adventures!

ONE

High School Reunion

When my good friend Sandy told me about Tim, I knew we had to pay him tribute. The desire and the intensity came from deep within. Could I explain it? I simply knew I had to follow my gut feeling. I'm glad I didn't anticipate the hazards.

Tim, Sandy and I first met in grade seven at Glenbrae Middle School in Hamilton. We went through middle school and two years at Glendale Secondary together.

September always rolled around faster than I ever wanted it to. September 1971 was no exception. I sat in a desk, which would become my designated seat in homeroom class. Sandy, who was to become a lifetime friend, took a desk in the row to my left and directly beside me. I didn't say much, but only because this was the first day of school and my first day at yet another school.

Sensing Sandy's shyness, I waited a day or two to introduce myself. Although I don't remember our first conversations I am absolutely certain I did the majority of the talking and probing to keep the conversation going. I often marvel at how opposites attract.

Besides family, Sandy is the only one to put up with me for more than 40 years. She probably deserves a medal.

Back in about 1998, Sandy called me to inform me that Glendale was having a reunion which included a 25th anniversary celebration for our graduating year. Though I didn't graduate from Glendale I attended school for almost four years with the class. Almost four years was the longest my family stayed in one area. Actually we physically moved twice during my Glendale years, but the moves were in the same school district. Our many moves were probably the reason why I didn't have many close friends.

The reunion or the thought of going to a reunion was somewhat nerve-racking. Would I remember people? Those high school years seemed a long way back. Would people remember me? With nervousness and excitement tossing around in my belly, I agreed to go.

Still on the telephone, Sandy and I began throwing people's names back and forth, wondering where they were in their lives. We enjoyed discussing old boyfriends and reminisced about regular lunchroom friends. We had been creatures of habit, sitting in the same place, with pretty much the same people lunch after lunch. Most of us found a fit, while some struggled to be accepted, or at least perceive to be accepted.

That's how Tim's name came up.

I had known Tim since grade seven. We were in the same homeroom. He sat several rows to the left and behind me. Not only were we in the same homeroom, but we shared several other classes as well. Math was one of those classes. I loved math—math and sciences, figuring things out, keeping my mind working. On the other hand, I struggled with English and French, the languages. (Yet now, as I type out this chapter, I earn a living communicating, speaking, teaching, training and facilitating, as well as a natural health care practitioner. I become energized standing in front of a group, as I watch faces light up when they catch something that will help them unlock their best. This has always been part of me.)

Tim struggled with math. Tim struggled with life. Now as I describe Tim some might think I am judging him. That is not my intent. My heart was always somewhat sad for him. Right from the beginning I knew Tim just wanted to be accepted. He was tall; he was probably the tallest person in the class. His physique made him different than the rest of the class. He had the longest arms, legs and fingers I have ever seen. I am sure he was quite aware of his physical differences and thus tried to adjust for his height by rounding his shoulders as he walked and slouching when he sat in his desk. Those one-size-fits-all desks didn't help. I was about a foot shorter than Tim and I remember feeling cramped in my desks.

Tim had shoulder-length straight thin hair. Shoulder-length hair was common back in the mid-seventies. Uncommon was the colour of Tim's hair. He had the blondest blond, almost white but not albino, hair in the whole school. He tried fitting in, but everything about Tim stood out. His appearance was different and everyday his classmates made sure he knew. The guys were verbally and physically cruel. The girls would stare and laugh at Tim from their little huddles. All this negative attention robbed Tim of any self-esteem.

I knew Tim had a crush on me. In fact the whole class knew Tim had a crush on me. It was grade seven; I didn't want Tim to have a crush on me. To be honest I was just trying to fit in and be accepted myself. I was cordial to Tim but didn't go out of my way to be more than just courteous.

One day as our math teacher—who if I remember correctly, was also our homeroom teacher—was handing back graded math tests. I can picture the room and where we were seated. As he handed Tim his test he commented, "If you don't do better you will fail this year." Then he added, "You should ask Diane to help you with your math." Just imagine the next ten seconds of comments from a class of grade sevens. I was embarrassed. Tim was embarrassed. To this day I puzzle over the insensitivity of that teacher.

Being who I am, I did tutor Tim. In fact he came to my home several times so I could help him with his math. His math grades improved, and I was privileged to get to know him somewhat better. But, Tim's self-esteem didn't improve. By high school he was looking for anyone, or any group to allow him to belong, whatever the cost.

Glendale, like most high schools, had a social structure. The way-out group—drugs, parties, four-inch platform heels, leather, knee-high boots, tight jeans, long hair, usually smokers—this group was not very large compared to the other groups, but this clique was different and stood out because it was so different. By grade ten these individuals had "accepted" Tim, or so he thought. Those of us who looked at the situation from the outside knew they hadn't accepted him at all, but were using him for laughs and their own enjoyment. I remember talking with Tim for a moment in a school hallway. I told him, "You're better than what you are doing."

Tim got into drugs. On many a Monday morning stories flew through school about Tim getting wasted on drugs or—more often—on a combination of drugs and drinking. We heard about the dangerous things he did in a drunken stupor. This escalated Tim's feeling of acceptance. People were talking about him. People that had never talked to Tim before were coming up to him in the halls and patting him on the back, "Way to go man." One time, totally dissipated, he let someone shave the top of his head in the shape of a light bulb.

When I moved, yet again, in the middle of grade ten, I lost track of Tim.

"So what happened to Tim?" I asked Sandy as we discussed the reunion.

There was a long pause on her end, "Diane, he passed away, I thought I told you." I'm sure I would have remembered if she had. She went on to say, "Yeah, he contracted AIDS and committed suicide."

In that moment I knew in my heart I had to do something. Immediately a plan formed. I had to write a memorial for him and the memorial would have to be at the reunion. As I sat down in front of my keyboard a poem welled up inside me. The words flowed from my mind to my fingertips and onto my computer screen. This was beyond human. It was powerful. Physically I felt different inside as I typed the poem. This was not just any poem but a very poignant poem about Tim. The words were about how people used him. People didn't understand his heart. I described his appearance and linked it to our blindness. I wish I still had that poem today but I don't. I remember reading it to Sandy. We both, she and I, knew it was good and would be a credit to Tim.

Next, I called Glendale Secondary School. The person who answered was a kind, gentle sort. She felt my pain and understood my desire to honour Tim. She went out of her way to dig out an old yearbook, find his class picture, blow it up, frame it and place this photo beside the poem I had written. She set up this display at the school.

All was well in my soul.

As Sandy and I went through the halls of Glendale Secondary School on the Friday evening of our class reunion we searched everywhere for Tim's picture and my poem. We finally found it. The secretary I had contacted had come through. True to her word, Tim would be remembered.

I only attended on the Friday evening of the reunion. I enjoyed seeing old friends, remembering their names and being remembered. I was oblivious that this weekend was to be a step in adventurous living, a step toward being able to walk in trust, not totally understanding, but trusting and acting on that gut feeling.

Monday morning the phone rang. I recognized the voice as belonging to the secretary at Glendale Secondary School. She struggled for words, but eventually told the wretched tale. She had just been on the phone with Tim's family. They were not happy. As she understood it, Tim's family had not seen him for many years. She was not sure how many years but it was more than a few. They knew he was dying but they did not know that he had passed away. When they saw his photograph and read the poem on Saturday afternoon at the reunion, naturally they became upset. They had not had any contact with him for a very long time and it took them two days of searching to determine if in fact he had passed away.

It got better or worse, depending on your point of view. Tim hadn't passed away. His life partner had passed away. Yes, Tim had AIDS and was dying, but he was still alive, not well, but alive.

I sank to the floor with the phone still next to my ear. I could hear the concern and strain in the secretary's voice. She had trusted me. She went above and beyond: looking for his photo, framing it and displaying his photo with the poem. I felt foolish. I felt worse for her. The school board had received the initial complaint from the family. They had contacted her. Her authorities expressed concern that she had not validated the information before doing what she did. I could see their point. Although my heart was in the pit of my stomach, she was on the hook for what we had done. I profusely apologized. What else could I do?

For what seemed like hours I sat on the floor crying. What had I done? I couldn't even imagine how Tim's family felt. Even though they had disconnected themselves from Tim, I am sure somewhere in their hearts they still cared for him.

And the secretary, how could I help her?

Another question bothered me more. Was that overwhelming gut feeling, that sense that I had to do this, that power thing that happened to me when I was typing the poem legitimate or not? It felt so right. Where did all those words come from? I knew they did not come from me. What had come over me? Something came over me! It felt so right to honour him. I was confused. Could I ever trust that feeling? How could such a knowing, such good intentions turn so sour?

These thoughts haunted me for that week. I replayed the secretary's words over and over. In my mind I repeatedly revisited the day I had typed the poem, remembering how easily the words flowed, recalling the overwhelming power and strength in the doing. There were no answers. There was no clarity.

Mid-afternoon at the end of that week after that phone conversation with the secretary, I was up in the bedroom when the phone rang again.

I didn't recognize the male voice, but his first sentence caught my full attention. My heart, my breath, everything in me seemed to stop in attention. The voice said, "Hello Diane, it's Tim." I felt my legs slip out from under me. The bed softened my landing as my legs gave way and my bottom hit the side of the bed then slide gently to the carpet where I landed with my back resting on the side of the mattress.

Generally I am not lost for words. This time was an exception. I muttered, "I'm so sorry for the problems I caused. I want you to know I had good intentions..." Tim stopped my rambling, to assure me everything was okay.

He said, "What you did was one of the nicest things anyone has ever done for me." (As I write this, I realize I will hear these very words again, later in my life.) I could hear Tim was being honest and sincere; he wasn't just trying to make me feel good. Tim expressed gratitude for the time I helped him with math and that I said "hi" to him in the halls at school, when others ignored him.

Tim had acquired the copy of the poem from the school. He read me some of the words. "That's how I felt," he said. "How could you possibly know this?" I was asking myself the same question. I didn't have an answer.

As we continued to talk, the heaviness of my past week dissolved. Tim explained how years of non-acceptance had scarred him. He met his friend who became his life partner and that was the first time he felt accepted. His family somewhat disowned him after high school. Then they totally disowned him when he adopted a gay lifestyle. He and his family—parents and siblings—had not seen each other for many years. I could hear the pain in his voice as he spoke of those many years.

When his siblings saw his photo and read my poem the words stung. I had written the poem lambasting some of the students at

Glendale when in fact those very words touched a raw spot in family members. That poem opened them to healing their relationship with Tim. In fact Tim was going to have Sunday supper with his family, something that had been missing in his life for a very long time. Tim knew he was dying. He was open and realistic about it. He told me his medication helped him somewhat, but it was only a matter of time.

I haven't spoken to Tim since that telephone conversation. I don't know if he is still alive. I said he could call me again if he liked, but he hasn't. I asked for his number but he didn't share that with me and I didn't push him—he had already gone through a very emotional week.

Tim relieved any further anxiety I may have felt for the secretary. He assured me his family had contacted the school board, letting them know all was well, that they very much appreciated what the secretary had done for their family.

As for me, the confusion I went through for one week was well worth the final outcome. This episode has given me the courage to continue to follow that gut feeling, that prodding, that overwhelming knowledge that I really need to do something. The experience of writing the poem has taught me to trust that feeling. More importantly when I get that power sensation (I'll call it that for now), I know that something awesome will happen. When, is not always for me to know, but trusting and believing with every fibre that something will happen has grown to be part of my daily life.

What a difference a week can make.

TWO

Wray's Message

As mentioned in the introduction, physically and emotionally I went through a very rough eighteen months during my late thirties. After every possible test including a not-so-nice muscle biopsy, the medical world advised I would have to learn to live with the pain. They didn't know what was wrong with me except that my muscle fibres were not being held together, thus I had no strength to use my legs and arms. My legs were far worse than my arms. The prognosis: get ready for a lifetime in a wheelchair. I cried as I saw my life as a professional photographer—a source of joy, and my income—slipping away.

My savings were useful, but wouldn't last forever, so I began scouting for another income. In the late nineties the economy was good, people were planning for their future and many financial companies were training individuals to become financial consultants. This could work: I excelled at math, and as a photographer had gained plenty of experience dealing with people. A career as a financial consultant would involve my mind, so I could do it without having to rely on my body. This seemed a good fit.

It was a great fit. I breezed through my examinations in insurance and mutual funds. In no time I became a branch manager. As a branch manager, I was able to recruit people just as I had been recruited. I trained, mentored, double checked and signed their paperwork and, yes, just as in real estate or other commission careers I received a percentage of the commission on each transaction.

Joanne was one of my recruits. She answered an ad I ran in the Hamilton Spectator. During her training she mentioned she had a connection with someone in a fairly high position with a union in Hamilton. I have come to realize, it's not so much what you know but who you know, or who knows who.

Joanne was able to make an appointment to see her acquaintance and as her trainer and mentor I went with her to that appointment. This acquaintance recognized the information we presented as important and valuable to union members. He passed our names up to the head of the union, thus we presented our information to this man as well. The union head agreed our information was valuable.

We were at the right place at the right time. Unbeknownst to us, the union was going through some changes and was looking for exactly what we had to offer. Everything was lining up perfectly. It turned out that the president of the Hamilton union was also the head of the presidents of all the provincial union representatives. This was bigger than we could have imagined.

Anyone in sales will tell you a majority of deals are sealed at social events; it's just the paperwork that gets done in the office. There is much socializing and meeting various people with authority before signing on the dotted line.

That said, Joanne and I were asked to attend a golf tournament six hours north of Hamilton. Many provincial union heads would be attending, as well as some higher-ups from the United States. We needed to be at this event. Picture this: more than 100 union people, all men, and two women, Joanne and myself.

The union head in Hamilton highly recommended we participate by golfing on a team. They were playing best ball. Feeling slightly intimidated as she had never golfed, Joanne chose not to play. I had golfed but would not consider myself a golfer, barely a hacker. I did however own golf clubs. My husband presented me with golf shoes for the occasion. I thought my baseball shoes would do, but he didn't think so.

Joanne and I gave ourselves extra travel time as my muscle condition required many stops along the way. If I sat for long periods of time, my muscles would cramp painfully and tears would flow. I always tried to read my body to prevent this unsightly ordeal.

We finally arrived, booked into our hotel room and unpacked. According to the agenda we were due at Wray's house for a barbeque that evening. The golf tournament would take place the next day.

Wray was both host and cook at the exclusive barbeque where we met some twenty union executives. Dinner was great; the company enjoyable; and we were getting to know the people we needed to know.

At the tournament the next day, the union head from Hamilton, two other executives and I became a golfing foursome. Joanne tagged along in her own golf cart. I was grateful to be playing best ball and to be hitting consistently straight, not far, but straight. Several times we used my ball because it was the only one we could find. I didn't do badly on the greens either. It must have been the new golf shoes. The union executives were impressed and I gained a new level of confidence.

Back at the clubhouse after the game I was physically exhausted. I certainly would not have been able to do the course without the golf cart.

I had an hour to get much-needed rest before dinner. As all the social interaction was happening on the clubhouse patio, I headed for a quiet porch overlooking a hilly wooded area at the opposite side of the club. I didn't want to sit, so I walked down the front steps over to the wooden railing which fenced off the hilly wooded ravine. Wray found me there leaning on the top rail gazing out.

Now, Wray was probably in his early fifties—nice personality, well-mannered and affable. During our conversation he looked at me and the colour left his face. His eyes grew large and he just stared at me.

"Wray, are you all right? Wray what is going on?" I had to ask a number of times.

Awestruck, Wray eventually spoke, "Oh my God, I had a dream about you the other night. You are wearing exactly what you were wearing in my dream."

In most such situations a woman might be prone to think, "That's an original line," but I knew Wray wasn't making a pass. It wasn't that type of conversation. He genuinely had a dream and he thought I was in it. He repeated, "Diane I really did have a dream about you and you are wearing exactly what you wore in my dream." Wray continued, "I was to give you a message from God, but I can't remember the message."

I thought he was going to cry right then and there. He meant what he was saying; I could see the sincerity in his eyes; he was seriously upset that he couldn't remember the message.

His "I have a message from God" piqued my interest. This was definitely not a come-on. I felt perfectly safe standing there with

Wray, my curiosity aroused, waiting for his memory to kick in. We chatted about anything and nothing. I assured him he would remember if it was important.

Then he remembered, "I had to tell you to go to the Toronto Airport Christian Fellowship and be healed."

I had never heard of the Toronto Airport Christian Fellowship (TACF) even though I lived in Dundas—Toronto was only an hour away. I certainly lived closer to the place than Wray. He described TACF from what he had heard since he had never been there himself. He said, "A revival has hit there… people are coming from all over the world to be 'touched.'" Wray used a lot of jargon I didn't understand. As the conversation continued I was wondering if he had been 'touched.' Our conversation was becoming uncomfortable; I was definitely in unknown territory. Thank goodness, the dinner bell rang; I could escape from this exchange.

I thanked Wray for the information and went in to join the others at dinner.

Joanne and I accomplished what we set out to do on this trip. We had met with the decision-makers. Now we were invited to join the heads of the provinces, top executives and their American counterparts at an international convention in Seattle, Washington. I was to make the presentation at the convention, as Joanne was not yet fully licensed.

As we drove home I didn't mention my conversation with Wray. Why would I? Joanne and I were excited about going to Seattle, and right then, exhausted and in pain, I was eager to be home, to be with my children and husband.

Home at last, I just wanted to relax. My daughter Kerina, not yet 10, loved to cuddle, so cuddle we did. As Kerina and I lay on the master bedroom bed cuddling and watching TV, a commercial came on, the strangest commercial I had ever seen. People were dancing and waving flags while music played and people clapped. The announcer kept saying, "Come catch the fire at Toronto Airport Christian Fellowship." My heart started to pound; I had never seen this commercial before. Kerina and I were watching a station that we normally watched, so why was I seeing this commercial now?

It got worse. For the next three weeks every time I watched TV, no matter what channel, there would be a commercial about TACF and *Catch the Fire*. It was freaky. The commercials were haunting me, "Come, come, come."

These commercials I had never seen before, about a place I had never heard of before my conversation with Wray, were getting to me. On one occasion when Kerina and I were curled up watching TV and a perplexing TACF commercial filled the screen yet again, I asked Kerina, "If mommy goes to this place, will you come with me? I can remember Kerina saying, "No. Those people look crazy."

After another week of torment, I couldn't stand it any longer. I informed Kerina she was coming with me. She was the only one I could force to come with me. I didn't have the courage or guts to tell anyone in my family, not even my husband, about what had happened to me at that golf tournament. My husband Randy understood I was searching for spiritual answers, so I didn't have to go into a long explanation about why I wanted to go to Toronto.

I don't know if I can adequately describe my perception of TACF when we arrived that Wednesday evening. *Nice building, parking lot was full*. Kerina and I went through the front doors, *looked normal so far*. There was a bookstore to the right. We walked past a greeting desk with information pertaining to upcoming seminars and events—*so far so good.* Then we entered the main room. I'd never been to a "church" that didn't have pews; this "church" had stacking chairs, and lots of them. There were TV cameras on platforms in several locations, a sound system booth and a huge front platform. The floor was carpeted throughout.

At the back of the room we noticed a group of people joined in a circle holding hands and laughing. I wasn't sure what they were laughing at, but the oddness led me to grasp Kerina's hand a little tighter. I'm not sure whether I was holding her hand to protect her or to gain some of her strength. We found seats a few rows from the back, definitely not close to the front of the room as we might want to get out in a hurry. Finally the music began. They had a worship band; to be honest they had a great worship band. But, I was not comfortable with all the people dancing, clapping and waving flags. *What was with these people dancing and waving flags?* I had never seen anything like it, except of course on those irritating commercials.

Music, music, the music seemed to go on forever and finally a man got up to speak. Blah, blah, blah, blah, blah, prayers, announcements and then I heard, "On Wednesday nights we don't do healings. I had prepared a message for tonight...."

Oh great! Yeah right Wray, you heard God tell you to tell me to come here and I would be healed, and they don't do healings on a Wednesday night.

I was getting ready to leave when the guy up front said, "...BUT during worship the Lord impressed upon me that we need to do healings tonight." He went on to say he was throwing his notes out for the evening and would do things the way the Holy Spirit wanted them done. This was followed by more words I didn't understand.

They also prayed and sang loudly in strange languages, no two of them sounded the same. *Weirdos*.

The guy up front would say things like, "If anybody has pain in their left shoulder, God wants to heal that. Come forward and be touched by the Holy Spirit's healing power." I could have sworn every nut-bar from around the world was in that room on that particular Wednesday night. People would go forward to the microphone up on the platform which served as a stage. The man would ask them where they were from. I can remember one lady from England—her accent confirmed she was indeed from England—went up for healing. I don't remember what she needed healing for, but I do remember her shaking and crying out as they prayed for her. Then she went limp and fell down, flopping around on the stage like a seal out of water. Oh, she wasn't the only one flopping about and doing other strange things. I had had just about as much circus entertainment as I could stand and felt I had been duped. I couldn't even imagine what Kerina was thinking about all this.

Then the guy at the front said, "There is someone in the audience who hasn't come up yet. They came here to be healed. They have a muscular issue, legs and arms but mostly legs. They need to come up." My heart started to pound. *Could it be true, God wanted to heal me. No way, I wasn't going up there. This was so phoney, but maybe not. Yes it was. This was ridiculous.*

Kerina said, "Mom that's you, you have to go up there." I let her know in no uncertain terms I was not about to go up there to make a fool of myself. I was sure this was an act. *This was staged and a cruel trick to play on people. I was smarter than this; I wasn't going to play their little game. I was staying put, right there in my seat, watching all those fools go forward and fall limp to the ground.*

I was certain there was some logical explanation for this display. I was looking around to see if there were fans blowing these people over. I didn't see any. *Must be magnets. Yes, there are magnets in the floor that somehow control their body movement.* This was the only other explanation I could invent. I had one word for this carnival: *phoney,* okay two words, *phoney baloney.*

Again the speaker appealed, "The person still hasn't come forward, legs, and arms, a muscular issue, come forward. It's your time to be healed." I couldn't believe my ears; again this announcer was describing my body. Kerina kept telling me, "Mom, go forward. Isn't that why we came here? Go mom, that's you they are talking about."

I couldn't go forward. *This was utterly stupid, beyond utterly stupid. Why had I come here? It was so obvious that this was phoney. Come on, who could believe this performance?*

Again the appeal, "The person hasn't come forward yet. You need to come forward."

By this time I was getting mad. *Okay, I will go forward and I will prove you wrong. I will expose your scam; nobody is going to make a fool of me.* I told Kerina to come up with me. (Yes, aren't I a brave one?)

Kerina said, "No mom, this is for you. You need to go up there, and I will stay right here and watch you."

Okay, I needed to get this over with. I crossed my arms in front of me, determined to prove them wrong. I am not sure who I was proving it to, but I was going to find those fans and magnets and they were not going to put me down.

My arms stayed crossed all the way up to as far as I made it, which wasn't even to the stage. I hit an invisible force that grabbed me, held me and gently laid me on the ground. I remember having absolutely no control of my body as I jerked about on that floor, but I distinctly remember not being afraid. I could hear everything around me, yet I couldn't see anything. Finally my body came to rest and a profound peace enveloped me. It took me several minutes, if not longer, to be able to pull myself together enough to get up. I felt different but didn't know what that difference was. I remember the heat that went through my body as I lay on the floor. A tingling heat is the best way to describe it.

I walked back to where we had been sitting. Kerina looked at me and with calm childlike faith said, "I guess you got healed."

I wasn't sure what had happened. I wasn't sure how I was going to explain this to Randy. Luckily by the time we arrived home Kerina had fallen asleep. I had to wake her up, and she was too tired to talk to anyone. Randy was also asleep. No questions were asked that night. The next day and thereafter everyone except me seemed to have forgotten that Kerina and I had even been out Wednesday evening. I didn't have to explain anything to anyone, which was fine with me.

Since then, I have come to learn that there are all types of physical healings. Some people have had complete instant healings that last and the illness never returns. Others have instant healings, but symptoms of the disease return or partially return at a later date. For me, I was immediately, partially, physically healed. My healing can be described as continuous. From that Wednesday on I had more physical strength and endurance, but more importantly I started on a path toward healing of the mind and soul. I have come to realize that we are comprised of three parts: mind, body and soul. We can work on healing the physical body, and some issues are all physical, but in most cases what is going on in the mind is intricately tied to wellness in the other two areas.

Now back to Joanne and the union. Joanne and I went to Seattle, made our presentation, and we were about to move forward overseeing the pensions and financial needs of union members across Canada and eventually the States, but these things were not meant to be.

In those days, financial consultants were technically self-employed but needed a sponsoring company. Every year sponsoring companies audited the offices under their umbrella. I shared my office with several other branch managers. During the annual audit I was pulled aside and questioned about my other involvements. At that time, a financial services consultant was not allowed to hold other licenses or occupations. Someone had mentioned to the auditor that they had heard me speaking to an audience about health and wellness. This was true; I was getting better and stronger every day. I had accepted several engagements to speak to different groups and audiences about taking control of their health. This had become my passion. It seemed head office saw this as possibly unacceptable. My licenses were suspended while an investigation took place. I was still receiving trailer fees and residual income but was not allowed to write new business. What I thought was my own business was in fact not in my control.

Head office in Toronto could not make a decision so they sent my case to head office in the States. Eventually, the ruling came back that I was not in violation of the "rules." They decided my speeches about health and wellness did not conflict with the business of financial services.

In the meantime with some helpful insight from my husband, I decided that since the sponsoring company seemed to need to be in control of more than the financial services part of my life, and since my passion was health and wellness, I needed to cut ties with them and follow my heart.

THREE

Orange Truck

In the fall of 2002 we began looking to purchase a new pick-up truck. Each month since the spring, we seemed to be spending more money on our 1990 GMC than it was worth. Yet, the idea of buying a new vehicle was somewhat overwhelming. The prices of vehicles, especially pick-ups, had taken an astronomical jump while we were obliviously driving around in our worn-out GMC. We were not mentally or financially prepared to shell out that much money.

We needed a pick-up—our life-style demanded it. A car wouldn't do. We had a minivan at one time and it wouldn't do: we camped; we trucked our mountain bikes; and the kids played hockey. We did not want to be in the same compartment with those stinky hockey bags on our sometimes long drives home from hockey games. Even a short trip home with a hockey bag can be unbearable.

After looking at every make and model, the Avalanche seemed like the only good fit for us. It had four doors, room for six and came with a fully extended truck bed. It also carried a steep price tag, a very steep price tag. Weeks and months went by as we searched and searched and kept coming back to the Avalanche.

One day I was driving our car along Hamilton's Main Street heading towards the Parkdale area when a decided peace settled over me. An inner voice indicated we could buy the truck. I felt that inner feeling I get when God is asking for my attention, heard a thought (a thought that was not my own) saying, "Put the truck on *don't-pay-for-a-year* and I will look after it. It will be okay."

Now, I personally am a very practical spender. Our family doesn't believe in using a credit card unless we actually have the money to pay the full balance when the statement arrives. We tried to instil this concept in our children as well. So, to make such a large purchase without any idea how we were going to pay for the truck at the end of the year was a big stretch. But, at this stage in my spiritual journey I was allowing myself to confidently trust that quiet peace that enveloped me and that creative inner voice that spoke thoughts into my mind. I was even able to share my confidence with my husband. When I arrived home that evening I told Randy what had happened and we agreed to buy the Avalanche. Thus by following another prompting we launched into another adventure.

The timing couldn't have been better as the old pick-up was having yet another challenge.

Back at the dealership, the salesman must have thought, "Here they are again." But, this time we were ready to make an offer and see what we could get for the old pick-up. After negotiating the price, we had to decide on the colour. When I asked Randy his preference, I was extremely surprised to find out he was thinking of an orange truck. All this time we had been looking at a black vehicle.

When Randy made up his mind, "Yes, let's get orange," the inner voice started talking to me again, "When Randy drives back and forth to work he will be doing spiritual warfare for Me." This seemed a rather strange message. For one thing Randy wasn't quite as enthusiastic in learning all the spiritual stuff that I was interested in learning. On the other hand, Randy would be driving back and forth from our home in Dundas on the west end of Hamilton to his work at Stelco in the east end of Hamilton.

So in the early part of 2003 we rode home in a newly acquired orange Avalanche and Randy drove that orange truck back and forth from Dundas to Stelco every workday.

In the meantime, I was on a steep learning curve about spiritual issues. I do not understand how I could have attended a variety of churches over the years since the time I was a young girl and not become aware of any of these things. Most Sundays I would be in church attentively listening to the message. I know I wasn't sleeping. Now I was growing in areas I had never even heard of before. One of these areas was intercession or prayer for the needs of others. As I read the newspaper, an issue would capture my attention so I would pray. I would pray about issues and for people whether I knew them or not. I simply knew I needed to pray for them. I also knew I was the one to pray about these things. This was not something to take to my pastor or friends so they could pray; I knew it was my privilege to pray for that person or situation.

This was specifically my privilege, not a prayer burden as some might call it. I was entrusted through spiritual prompting with the honour to pray for someone or something that possibly no one else was praying about. I believe these promptings were not mere coincidences or chance happenings. A relationship with God is a two-way adventure. The Holy Spirit prompted me to pray. At this stage I was discovering my relationship with the Holy Spirit, again a concept I didn't understand totally. I was realizing that to trust the sense brought on by the Holy Spirit is a high that no drug or alcohol could ever, ever produce. All these years going to church, hearing about the Trinity—Father, Son and Holy Spirit—did not give me even a clue about the beauty of this ultimate relationship.

By August 2004, prayer had become a daily part of my life. I wrote my prayers. There is no right or wrong way to pray. Writing my prayers worked for me. One day I read a newspaper article about financial trouble at Stelco. Now you would think since my husband worked at Stelco I would be worried about his job and our future, but that is not what had my attention: I was concerned for pensioners. Most pensioners were likely beyond being hired by anyone. How could they survive if something happened to their pension? Knowing that divorce is often due to financial issues, I felt I needed to pray for families, that the financial strain wouldn't tear them apart. So I prayed.

I didn't track just how long I prayed for pensioners, but I do know I shed a lot of tears.

Then I heard the gentle nudging voice, "It's not good enough that you privately pray for Stelco, you need to hold a citywide time of prayer for Stelco." The voice went on to give me the step-by-step organization for this citywide prayer. Of course it was entirely up to me whether to follow this plan. Initially, I wanted to get right on it. To me, a task-minded, goal-oriented person, the plan sounded quite reasonable, until I began thinking about reality.

I got on the phone to the senior pastor at the church we were now attending. After my bizarre, but healing experience at TACF, we had sought out a church where the unusual, supernatural things could be explained to us. We had found a place where we felt at home and were encouraged to grow and learn. I explained my prayer-time experience to my pastor. I told him about the instruction to hold a citywide prayer event, the step-by-step plan as well as my second thoughts. My senior pastor couldn't have been more supportive, encouraging and helpful in his suggestions.

In three days the whole event was organized—according to the step-by-step instructions as I recalled them. The very first step was to contact the faith and ethics reporter at the *Hamilton Spectator* to explain the citywide time of prayer to be held at Dundurn Park after the city's annual Labour Day parade. Hamilton, nicknamed Steel City, is a largely unionized industrial city. Every Labour Day the roads are closed as all the organized unions march in a parade ending at Dundurn Park. Yes, I called the *Spectator* first before I called anyone else. That was the first step in the plan. It wasn't my plan. I wasn't in charge of the outcome. All I had to do was follow the instructions. Some might call my blind faith naïve. It wasn't. Up until now, following the promptings always led to something positive. I simply believed everything would work out.

In three days, people from different churches and denominations joined the formal team of helpers for that day. A banner was printed, flyers were made and everything was in place. Even a sound system was available for the day. I had one minor detail to tie up. I needed to talk to my senior pastor about how he wanted to do the actual prayer time.

As I sat in his office reciting the details of the event I finally came to the part where I had slotted him to do the prayer. He looked at me with his trademark "silly" grin and said, "Diane I don't think I am the one that is suppose to pray. You got the message—it's you who has to pray."

He was saying this to a woman who had not yet grasped the etiquette of prayer. The words I heard people use in prayers weren't even part of my vocabulary. I was one who not so long ago had prayed, "Lord please forgive all those that didn't do what I asked them to do." Does that sound like a person who should take the microphone to pray in front of hundreds of people? No, definitely not.

I am not afraid of public speaking. I am actually one of those crazy people who get juiced when speaking in front of a crowd; the speaking in front of a crowd wasn't the issue. Clearly my issue was my inability to pray in front of people. I could say it like it is, but a suave grammatically correct, flowery prayer—my idea of a public prayer—was beyond my capability.

When my senior pastor, in all seriousness, told me I should be the one to pray, I wanted to call the whole thing off. My stomach flopped and then flipped and then flopped again. My heart began to race. I was rendered speechless—which rarely happens. My face screamed, "Are you out of your mind?" All colour drained from my body and my eyes opened up as wide as eyes could open. I stared at my pastor and squeaked, "There is no way!"

He looked at me, "Diane, you can do this. I know you can." In time I learned that he has a unique gift of encouragement. He is one of the few people I know who allow people to stretch and grow. He isn't threatened by growth, but actually encourages those around him to grow to their full potential.

I pleaded with him that day and for many days thereafter right up until he left for a holiday just prior to the Labour Day parade. He knew he wasn't to be the one to pray because he already knew he wouldn't be around on Labour Day. He did help me put my prayer on paper before he left.

Prior to Labour Day, the *Spectator* published an article about the prayer gathering. After reading the article Larry DiIanni, a city councillor, called me in support. His dad was a pensioner from Stelco, so this hit home for him.

On Labour Day 2004, Randy and I drove the orange Avalanche to Dundurn Park where the parade would end. We parked on the grass, erected the banner, and handed out flyers to all the volunteers to pass out as they walked the parade route. We set up the sound system and did a sound check.

Then we waited for the parade to finish. We waited for the moment when I would climb up onto the bed of that orange truck to do spiritual warfare by praying for Stelco.

As the people began to arrive at Dundurn Park as the parade wound down, I found myself behind a tree throwing up. With my stomach in a knot, shaking so bad inside I couldn't control my chattering teeth, I waited until the parade finished, then I climbed into the back of our orange truck, explained why we had gathered and asked people to join hands and bow their heads. Shaking with nervousness and downright fear, I took a deep breath then read my five-minute prayer.

I have been told the prayer was heard right to the other end of Dundurn Park, even though the sound system was not capable of projecting the sound that distance. Hundreds of people watched, listened or prayed along as I spoke into the microphone mounted on our orange truck. This was spiritual warfare.

There was also something else, a more personal matter, the Holy Spirit addressed that day. I'd been told years earlier that women could never lead in matters relating to God. Up until I did that prayer from the back of the truck, I had allowed that lie to hold me back by creating confusion within. I knew I was a leader and had leadership capabilities. Now I was beginning to grasp that He did have a perfect plan for me; now I was no longer confused about why He made me a woman *and* gave me leadership qualities; now I could be the woman he has made and use the leadership abilities He has given me. The lie no longer has a grip on me.

As the payment-free year on the truck was steadily winding down, Randy and I were still wondering how we would be able to settle our account. Then one evening in October upon returning home, we found a note from a real estate agent in our mailbox. She had a client who was interested in our home. Randy and I looked at one another; we had talked about moving. "Well, it's worth the phone call," we agreed.

After that one phone call, and one walk-through with the client, the agent presented an offer. Normally, the seller of a home pays commission to a real estate agent, but in this case we were selling the house with no agent working on our behalf. I made it clear to the buying agent that we would not be paying her a fee, but if she wanted she could be our agent in the purchase of another home and thus would be paid from that sale. She agreed.

Six weeks later we moved from our home in Dundas to a new place in Ancaster. We paid for the truck with the money we saved on commission fees and the equity we had gained on our home over three years. The cost of housing had increased so dramatically that we still had a good down payment on our next home. The truck was paid in full by the end of the year, and curiously, not by anything we initiated on our own. We were beginning to have a lot more trust and faith in "the promptings."

FOUR

Prayer at City Hall

As my 'God adventures' played out I saw a connection from one to the next. Threads of people, places and situations were weaving in and out of each individual adventure connecting into a larger pattern. Something I was prompted to do with no foreseeable result in one adventure would turn out to be the exact action necessary to kick-start the next. A person I'd be introduced to in one adventure, would be key in the next leg of my journey.

Prayer at city hall happened that way. A group of Christians from various denominations had the privilege of praying at Hamilton's city hall in council chambers for three hours every Thursday night for three and a half years. Yes, for three and a half years people gathered in council chambers where all the critical decisions were made for our city. How did this come about?

Remember City Councillor Larry DiIanni who supported the Stelco prayer gathering? Mr. DiIanni at the time of the prayer for Stelco, represented Ward 9 in Stoney Creek. In 2003 Councillor Larry DiIanni became the honourable Mayor Larry DiIanni of the City of Hamilton. The only councillor I personally spoke with during the prayer for Stelco at Dundurn Park was now the mayor of the city.

In December 2003 during one of my regular times of prayer and intimate reflection I had one of those *prompting* experiences. I knew I was to make an appointment with Mayor Larry DiIanni to discuss with him the need to have prayer for our city at city hall. By now I trusted the promptings and was confident enough to follow the "feeling." The results so far had been amazing. I felt I had absolutely nothing to lose.

Typically when you call to make an appointment with the mayor of a city, population 500,000, the first person you talk to screens you, then gives you the standard speech, "The mayor is very busy. I will pass the message to him and get back to you." That didn't happen. I called in December 2003 and I had an appointment January 6th 2004. I was beginning to see a power at work beyond anything Diane Elms could produce of herself.

On January 6th 2004 I met with the Honourable Larry DiIanni in his office at city hall in Hamilton Ontario. Conversation flowed naturally. I went straight to the reason why I had asked to meet. "Mayor DiIanni, this city needs to be covered in prayer."

"God only knows that this city needs prayer," he agreed.

"Yes, God knows. That is why he sent me." Where did that answer come from? It certainly surprised me when that flowed out of my mouth. Mayor DiIanni consented to look into the availability of council chambers to hold weekly Christian, non-denominational prayer gatherings for the city of Hamilton. He said he would connect with me in a week.

One week, then another week went by and nothing. I called the mayor's office once more. I felt the mayor had been sincere and the issue couldn't be with him. I was right. One of his top aides wasn't in favour of the mayor sticking his neck out for a prayer event. This aide made sure I understood he would get back to me when he felt like getting back to me.

During the third week of waiting for an answer, I received some material in the mail. I was expecting the material; I just wasn't expecting the profound effect this material had on me. As I watched this information video, I Timothy 2:1-4 commanded my attention. "Pray for those in authority." Was this a joke? I had never prayed for those in authority before. It hadn't crossed my mind to pray for them.

To be honest, the only time I had mentioned an authority's name was to slam the person. When our property tax bill arrived it never occurred to me to bow my head and say, "Oh dear Lord, thank you for those in authority who increased my property tax bill." No, I said things like.... well, I don't think I should repeat what I said. Truthfully, I never thought about this verse before and, again, had never heard the verse taught or discussed in a church message.

The verse goes on to say, we need to pray for them so that *we* can live in peace and harmony. I am paraphrasing, but that is what it means. Can you grasp that? It is our responsibility to pray for those in authority so *we* can live in peace. This is very, very specific direction for living.

Then I read 2 Chronicles 7:14 which outlines the reoccurring theme in my adventures thus far: be humble, pray and be healed.

I knew by the feeling I was getting that I was going to be prompted to do something that I probably didn't want to do. I was right. The prompting was to write an email to send to all the current councillors and Mayor DiIanni asking for forgiveness for not praying for them before. I was being asked to humble myself.

The opposite of 'humble' is 'proud.' In other words I was being asked to get rid of my pride and ask *those* people—those people in authority, some whom I personally knew from organizations that I belonged to—for forgiveness. Wasn't it bad enough that people already thought I was *way out there*? And now, I was being prompted to ask those people for forgiveness. I use the word 'prompted' because whether I did it or not was my choice. I didn't have to send that email. I knew that. I knew I could take the easy way out. I also knew I wouldn't be comfortable with my decision if I decided to take the easy way out. But, to send an email asking for forgiveness, that was too much.

Personally I wanted some people to ask me for forgiveness for things they had done and said to me. But no, I was being asked to ask for forgiveness. Somehow, this didn't seem fair. Wasn't a certain amount of pride good for a person? I would be in a meeting with a few of those people in the next week or so. How could I face them after sending them an email asking for forgiveness? I would become the butt of their jokes. I knew them. I knew their personalities. I had been in a room listening to their cutting sense of humour at another's expense. Their comments never seemed very humorous to me. Yet these were the people in authority whom I was supposed to look up to and now pray for and, worse, ask for forgiveness.

This was torture. I was being tortured. Why me?

I felt as if my dignity was going to be stripped away. How could I hold my head up at the next meeting? I felt that if I sent that email I would lose respect. No longer the poised, confident woman, I would never again be able to strut into a room with these people. I would be considered a sheepish, weak female. I had worked hard so people understood they couldn't—or wouldn't even try—to pull a fast one on me. I held my ground, pulled my own weight and in fact probably tried harder and pulled more than my fair share of weight on any team project. I needed my pride, damn it. I needed them to know I was a force to be reckoned with, not some female weakling asking for forgiveness. Aaaahh, the pain!

This was one of those times when prayer became a crying, sobbing, screaming one-way conversation. It wasn't fair. Why did I have to ask for forgiveness? I was just an ordinary citizen who, until now, didn't know those verses existed. What about all ministers in the city of Hamilton? Why didn't they have to ask for forgiveness? They should be the ones asking for forgiveness. They were paid to do that sort of thing. Had I not done enough?

I spent hours tossing and turning this prompting until I was tired and exhausted. The prompting never changed and I still had a choice.

At one o'clock in the afternoon on January 28th I pressed the send button of my email asking all the councillors and the mayor of the city of Hamilton for forgiveness for not praying for them before.

I also called my senior pastor to tell him of the day's events and what I had just done. I was exhausted. Emotional experiences certainly can be draining.

A little later that day, the email notification sounded off on my computer. I swivelled my desk chair around to my keyboard. I had just received an email from the facilities help desk at city hall. "We have been contacted by the mayor's office to book space for you and your events. Please contact our department to confirm dates and times."

I immediately called their office. It was now 4:15 and the office closed at 4:30. My contact at the facilities help desk was very accommodating. She emailed me forms to fill out. We confirmed every Thursday evening from then until the end of 2004 from 7 to 10 p.m. as a time of prayer and worship with a focus on praying for those in authority and for businesses in the City of Hamilton.

Thus, Prayer at City Hall launched.

The next morning I had a long and exciting conversation with my senior pastor. We discussed a safe and appropriate format for prayer. I needed to be sensitive to the differing styles of prayer from the various denominations. This time of prayer was to bring unity among different denominations who normally didn't gather together.

I didn't even object to leading the prayer times. I was becoming more comfortable with praying in public. If anyone had told me previous to February 2004 that I would be leading an interdenominational prayer gathering in council chambers at city hall in Hamilton, I would have said that was impossible.

My senior pastor and I felt we had all the details in place: date, time, format, team members, worship arrangement and location. The only thing missing was the publicity. How would we get this information to the masses? To come, people had to know about it. We didn't have a budget nor did we want to collect or raise money to get this thing going. After almost an hour on the phone we felt confident the Lord would work out our publicity dilemma.

Before I could put the phone down, it rang and flashed *Hamilton Spectator*. I was thinking, 'That's odd, why would the *Hamilton Spectator* be calling me?'

"Hello. Is Diane available?"

"Yes, this is Diane."

"It's Sharon Boase, the faith and ethics reporter from the Hamilton Spectator, just wondering what your thoughts are on

Stelco's announcement that they have just applied for bankruptcy protection. Do you think your time that you gathered at Dundurn Park on Labour Day was a waste?"

"Absolutely not. Now you are really going to see God at work. When most people give up hope, God can really shine." Again, I just shook my head and thought, 'Where did that comment come from?' I went on to explain how I had just received confirmation that we were given permission to meet in council chambers every Thursday evening starting in February.

Well, I am sure you have already put two and two together. The *Hamilton Spectator* ran the interview the very next day advertising the beginning of prayer at city hall. All the details were looked after with no budget needed. It is always amazing to see what happens when you follow through with a prompting.

Prayer at City Hall began in February 2004 and ran until the city hall building closed for extensive renovations three and a half years later. We as a team knew the time had come to end our prayer gatherings. During those three and a half years we prayed for businesses, including Stelco, current events and especially for all of those in authority: politicians, chief of police, fire chief, and superintendent of education. Many different denominations were represented during that time and we all knew we were in the right place at the right time.

In February 2005, I had the opportunity to introduce myself to Courtney Pratt, the chief executive officer of Stelco. He didn't recognize my name, but he did recognize what I represented. He thanked me for the emails that I sent to him on a regular basis—emails encouraging him and letting him know there were people praying for him and for Stelco.

In December 2005 Stelco was able to work out a deal and pulled out of bankruptcy protection. One of the main issues that had been of tremendous concern throughout the bankruptcy protection was the protection of pensions. The final deal protected pensions.

FIVE

Army Boots

So far each of my adventures has a tangible outcome. The reason I was prompted to do what I was prompted to do is evident for all to see. Tim's family reconnected with him; Wray's message lead to my healing; the truck was completely paid for and used in spiritual warfare; and prayer at city hall was awesome in so many ways. In each case I have a rationale to measure or qualify my seemingly illogical actions.

I like rational results. When I repeat an adventure to someone, I am greatly comforted by my ability to justify my actions. As a speaker I have shared my adventures with numerous audiences. I notice the expression in their eyes and on their faces. (*Okay, let's take a step back from this weirdo. What is this lady on? This stuff doesn't happen.*) Knowing I have a tangible outcome helps me handle those looks. When I share the outcome, the incredulous looks are replaced by looks of acceptance. Amazement replaces scepticism. I become credible.

But, not all my adventures end rationally or have a result I completely understand.

Prayer at City Hall started in February 2004. Committed team members joined and shared the load. Fran was one of those team members. I could bounce ideas off Fran. One problem: she was usually prompted to agree with the outrageous things I was being prompted to do and always encouraged me to follow through.

Sometimes I wished she would give me reasons not to do those things. For, even with all the positive outcomes I had already experienced, following the promptings wasn't my natural inclination. I am human. I appreciate being accepted and respected. I want to be normal, or at least, perceived to be normal.

In the summer of 2004 Fran and I grabbed a coffee and went to Sam Lawrence Park overlooking the heart of the city. Sam Lawrence was a former mayor of the city of Hamilton. He was known for the position he took when Stelco went on strike back in 1946. At that time he took an uncommon stand and actually joined the strike marches, picketing with the citizens of the city of Hamilton for better wages, safety and security. Most political figures tend to sit on the fence or sway towards big business, but not Sam Lawrence. He actually became known as Mr. Labour.

As Fran and I drank our coffee and chatted I shared a prompting I had been getting lately. It was a ridiculous prompting which made no sense at all. I even laughed as I told her I felt I was being prompted to buy a pair of army boots. Fran, being Fran, said, "Well go ahead and buy them." Nothing was too absurd for Fran.

Well, even with her encouragement I did not run out to buy a pair of army boots, although I knew where to get them. In Hamilton we have a long-standing army surplus store on Ottawa Street. As I had lived only a block away from this store at one point in my childhood, I was somewhat familiar with the place. In my mind this army surplus store only sold second-hand items. Not true, but that's what I thought at the time of the ridiculous prompting.

So after considering this prompting from every rational angle, I placed the issue on a back burner and conveniently forgot about it. Only, somehow this army boot prompting seemed to be more important than I could imagine.

That July, a friend and I went to a four-day camp retreat in Hermon, New York, an eight hour drive from home. I attended the retreat for sheerly selfish reasons—I wanted to get recharged. I had been giving and giving, people were taking and taking, and I needed some time for me. I truly enjoy giving but we all need time to recharge the batteries. I thought this retreat would be a place for me to relax and read.

To be honest I was in an agitated, negative mood when I arrived at the retreat centre. I preferred to be left alone which is why I had chosen to come to a retreat. I assumed a retreat was for privacy and quiet meditation. I had never been on a retreat before and didn't know that at this retreat I would be expected to participate in a program or agenda.

On the second night of our stay, we attended the scheduled program held in a large, newly erected auditorium which looked to me like a big implement building. It suited the country setting. This building had a concrete floor with a carpeted area where the chairs were placed.

The guest speaker (I can't remember his name) had been speaking for about an hour. As he wound down his message he invited people forward for prayer, specifically those that wanted more boldness. Many went to the front. I did not. More boldness was the last thing I needed or wanted.

The speaker spent time with each individual person who went forward, praying specifically as he felt prompted. The number of people at the front wanting prayer continued to grow. I was perfectly content to stand at the back of this rather large building watching the activity.

Suddenly the speaker yelled out, "Hey you, the one at the back in the Port Dover sweatshirt." That would be me. "You need to come forward."

I yelled back at him, "It's okay, thank you. You have lots of people to pray for, and I'm good."

The speaker yelled out again, "No, you need to come forward. I have a message for you."

Everything within me screamed, "No not again." Honestly, I was embarrassed. He was calling me to the front ahead of all the waiting people who wanted his attention. I didn't ask for or want any of it. Everyone stared as I walked to the front of the building where the crowd was gathered.

He put one hand on my shoulder, looked me straight in the eye and said, "God has a plan for you. You are a general in God's army." He continued to say things to me that he could not have known. We had never met before. Some of the things he said were things that only I knew.

You would think that now I would remember the prompting to buy army boots, but I didn't.

Time passed and prayer at city hall continued every Thursday evening. One Thursday a new face joined us. She had come just early enough to have a short conversation with one of the greeters on the team. The greeter was Fran.

As I believe in punctuality, we made a point of starting promptly at seven thirty. During the three and a half years of prayer at city hall I can only remember a small handful of times we were tardy in getting started. This Thursday evening was not one of those tardy times. Fran did not have the opportunity to let me in on the conversation that had just taken place.

Prayer at City Hall had a loose structure which allowed for various individuals to participate during the evening. Fran was eager to share the conversation she had had with the new face. Fran introduced Marian. She then asked Marian to share why she had chosen to come.

A few nights previous to this, Marian had suddenly awakened from a sound sleep with the words, "join the army at city hall" running through her head. She went right back to sleep. Again she awoke. The words, "join the army at city hall," filled her mind. She repeated the words to herself, trying to comprehend, "join-the-army-at-city-hall." What was that about? Then she remembered a fascinating article she had read in the newspaper some months before about prayer happening at city hall. In her mind, prayer was a type of warfare. She concluded she was being asked to join those who prayed at city hall. So here she was.

Fran then reminded me about the army boots, but I wasn't ready to dig up that idea.

Six months after squelching the first army boot prompting, in December 2004 during my morning quiet time, I felt a particularly intense prompting to buy the army boots. I knew I had been given yet another opportunity to choose my direction. Would I be doing this?

This time I chose to at least investigate at the army surplus store. The thought of wearing second-hand boots was not appealing. I have a thing about wearing other people's shoes. Feet are sweaty and can be smelly. Compound my "thing" with the idea of wearing used army boots. No good could come of wearing another person's army boots. My brother had been in the armed forces serving overseas. I had a good idea about what those boots went through. I knew army boots were an ideal breeding ground for festering foot fungus. You can imagine my repulsion.

The sales clerk at the army surplus store asked if he could help me. I explained I was looking for a pair of army boots. He looked at me sideways. I guessed I didn't look like the type to come into this store to buy army boots. He questioned why I wanted the boots. I stuttered and stammered. I was not prepared to share a reason. He persisted.

Please, please why couldn't I get a sales clerk that didn't give a tinker's darn about why I wanted these boots?

"Are you going to be in a play?" asked the store clerk.

"No?"

"So, why do you want the boots? I need to know what you want them for because you don't want to spend a lot of money on a new pair if you don't really need a new pair."

My eyes lit up, "You have *new* army boots?"

"Yes, we do," responded the clerk. "They cost 150 dollars, while the used are anywhere between thirty and forty dollars.

"What size are you?" he asked.

Normally I would be seven and a half with a medium width but I learned that army boots don't come in a typical shoe size. I ended up being a 4F. The clerk checked the stock for a new pair of army boots in a 4F. There weren't any. Now I didn't have a choice, it had to be second-hand boots. How gross!

If truth be known, I didn't have an extra 150 dollars, so I wouldn't have been able to buy the new army boots anyway. To be really honest, I regretted spending the forty dollars on used army boots. I was not convinced this prompting had rhyme or reason. How could it?

The clerk continued to harass me for my purpose in buying the boots. I refused to share my ludicrous reason. I left the store, my pride somewhat intact. Arriving home I flung—I mean *flung*—that plastic bag containing those stupid army boots to the back of the bedroom closet.

The next day Randy and I visited my brother and his family. This is the brother who had served in the armed forces. As quietly as possible I asked my brother how to clean army boots. He slowly turned his head, raised one questioning eyebrow and asked, "Why?"

"Shh, shhhh, I don't want Randy to hear me. I had to buy a pair of second-hand army boots. I felt prompted."

I think I need to qualify something. Randy had never said I couldn't do the wild and crazy things I felt prompted to do, but many of these promptings resulted in a newspaper article. Thus Randy received his fair share of looks and questions from his friends and his co-workers at Stelco. I felt any information I shared with Randy was on a need-to-know basis and right now he didn't need to know that I had purchased a pair of army boots.

As my brother stood looking at me, I knew by the look on his face, he was recalling something. Then he said, "Wait a minute. The other day when I was cleaning the furnace room, I came across a pair of brand new army boots. I haven't got a clue how they got there. If they fit you, they must be meant for you."

We proceeded to the furnace room and, yes, the boots were a 4F. So where did those boots come from? I don't know, but I know God arranged it.

With extreme gratitude for not having to wear second-hand army boots, I retrieved the bag containing the used army boots from the depths of my closet and returned to the army surplus store where I received a full refund on my purchase.

From then on I wore army boots to prayer at city hall every Thursday evening and to other places as I felt led.

To this day, I don't fully comprehend why I needed to go through this adventure. I know in my heart that the army boots themselves had no power. I didn't feel any different with the boots on or without the boots on as I led prayer at city hall and at other events.

Possibly it was a lesson—a lesson on letting go of my pride. Maybe it was a lesson about trusting even with little details. Personally this made me realize that God my Creator took my feelings into consideration. I realized He really does care about me, all the way down to my feet. And, as pointed out to me, my army boots made a statement and created a physical picture of spiritual purpose. Yet, I can't pinpoint a tangible outcome—other than the creation of an opening for many conversations. I have to wonder what might have happened if instead of waiting six months, I had chosen to be obedient when I first received the army boot prompting.

SIX

Barton Street

Not until I received inquiries from Western Canada, the United States and the United Kingdom, did I realize the impact of obeying the Barton Street prompt. The inquiries began after sharing about our Barton Street adventure on *Listen Up*, a half hour weekly television program exploring news and current affairs from a Christian perspective. *Listen Up* is broadcasted from coast to coast in Canada, on several American networks and on the internet. Upon watching the program, others wanted to do what we did. Yes, the influence of obedience to this particular prompting spread well beyond our local businesses.

At the time, we didn't realize our handful of people carrying out a simple task would have international impact. We were simply focussed on Barton Street, which had once been the economic heartbeat of Hamilton, but was now a seedy shadow of its former self.

In February 2005, I was having my usual coffee and early morning conversation with God, whom I picture as three beings in one: God the Father, Jesus and Holy Spirit. I knew a prompting was coming. I physically notice the shift in my body when I am about to have an intimate connection. God is always with me and never leaves, but this physical shift in awareness is my signal to pay attention. This particular prompting from God was to gather a team and walk down Barton Street, going into every business to assure the individuals in each establishment that people would pray for them. As I understood the prompting, the team was to go into every business, asking for prayer requests.

Those prayers would then be taken to the people praying at city hall on Thursday evenings. The requests would be prayed for at city hall and could be taken back to the various home churches. The home churches could then also pray for the businesses and people on Barton Street.

As always, I shared my prompting with my senior pastor, and as usual he thought what I had been prompted to do was a great idea.

The core team at city hall readily agreed to take on the venture. That didn't mean the core team would necessarily be part of the team walking Barton Street. They simply unanimously agreed the prayer requests could be brought to the Thursday night gatherings. Praying for the specific businesses' prayer requests would fit perfectly into the *Prayer at City Hall* vision to pray for Hamilton businesses, as well as for those in authority.

I wasn't at all concerned about where and when to start the project. From experience I trusted the details would fall into place. A further prompting surely would come.

Sure enough, in April of that spring I understood exactly where and when to begin. We were to visit every business on Barton Street, from Gage in the east to Locke in the west. Curiously, we were to begin at Beechwood and Gage, which wasn't on Barton Street, but located one block south. This instruction seemed odd since not only was that address not on Barton, but we were almost sure Beechwood and Gage was a residential corner.

Our plan was to break Barton Street into four sections. Our goal would be to visit each business three times a year. We would keep it simple: introduce ourselves, ask for prayer requests, and let it be known people would be praying for them. We would leave a letter explaining our unfettered offer to pray with a list of contacts should they have further requests.

Our intent was not to interrupt the business day. We did not want to create a scene or scare away customers. We also made a point of not dressing like salespeople. We didn't want to be perceived as coming in under false pretence. Personally I liked wearing business casual and my army boots.

Two people took the north side of Barton Street. The other two visited the businesses on the south side of the street. As a team we used common sense when entering businesses such as massage parlours, a strip club, the liquor store, and an occult shop. For instance we would not send a male into strip clubs or massage parlours. Common sense and prayer worked well.

The first day out, plans in place, letters in hand, we had two teams ready to go. Together we all walked to our starting point at the corner of Beechwood and Gage. To our pleasant surprise there was a business on that corner, *Sutton and Son*, a small appliance repair store. As the others waited outside, I walked up to the counter, introduced myself to the owner and handed him the letter I intended to leave. I told him people would be praying for his business and I asked him if he had any specific prayer requests. He looked at me stunned. I will never forget his reply.

"Yes, you could pray for our staff. One of our staff members just committed suicide. We're only a small business here and we are pretty tight with our employees. This has really hit us hard." He went on to explain the circumstances. I assured him we would all be praying for him and his employees. I pointed at my contact information on the letter suggesting he contact me if he felt so inclined.

Out on the street the team eagerly awaited my report. With mixed emotions I repeated the details of the tragedy. The team was in awe. *God really did care about every situation in our city.*

For me, this incident confirmed my prompting. The visit to *Sutton and Son* was a long needed personal assurance by my Father. Sending our team specifically to this small appliance repair store to show a few people He cared about them in their time of pain was plainly and simply love at its finest. I was beginning to understand God's love, a love I knew so little about and constantly desired.

I recorded the business name *Sutton and Son* in my notebook along with the date, owner's name and prayer request—an accurate record to be shared on Thursday evening at *Prayer at City Hall*. Don kept a similar notebook for the businesses he and his partner visited.

Don was amazing. He was literally a right-hand man. Age did not stop him. Still in his prime, several years beyond eighty, Don was totally committed to *Prayer at City Hall* and walking Barton Street. Wherever Don went, he left that place a better place.

Historically, Barton Street was at the core of Hamilton's economic development. In its heyday this street boasted thriving businesses of all kinds. Time had not done justice to the distinctive buildings, now with boarded windows and for-sale signs posted. Some days, deep sadness enveloped me as I walked past building after building, remembering better days on this street.

For a year and a half, Don and I consistently walked Barton Street. Often others would join us—people from different churches, different denominations, men and women, young and old. That is what made walking Barton Street so effective and allowed the business owners and store clerks to trust us.

On our first trip down Barton Street, store owners, managers, and staff would ask, "What's in it for you?"

"Nothing!" we would say. That was the beauty of this venture. No one on the team attended a church in the immediate area. The business owners, managers and staff took note.

"So why are you doing this?" they wondered.

"To let you know people are praying for you," we would reply. Their faces expressed doubt. At first the store owners, managers and staff did not believe us.

Some asked, "How much does this cost?" They wanted to know how much we were charging. I found that troubling. Is that what the general population thought? Did they believe Christianity to be about asking for money? Our team soon came to realize many people thought "the church" was all about money, money and give me more money.

It occurs to me they may have come to this conclusion watching TV evangelists. Yes, TV evangelists need cash to run their programs, but I personally have a hard time watching expensively dressed ministers flashing jewellery, asking for money. Prosperity is good and everyone needs to earn an income, but the blatant over-the-top continual appeal for funds turns many people away. The people on Barton Street taught me a lesson on the general perception of church as a money-hungry institution.

On the whole, the institution of the church has failed. Of course there are some exceptions. The exceptions focus on teaching the truth, the whole truth, not self-serving bits and pieces. Most important these churches teach about the relationship with our Heavenly Father. Church should be about relationship, without feeling shame, guilt or coercion. Relationship happens in the heart and can take a long time to fully develop. The relationship is based on trust. It's hard to trust the Father when some of those representing Him on earth have not been trustworthy. Ultimately the relationship is with Him from above and it has to come from each person's heart.

Some days while walking Barton Street, listening to the comments, I would become saddened by what the general public thought of God. God had us there for a reason.

The owner of *Ever Convenience* asked, "Why you come today? This is really important." It turned out he had been robbed the night before. He was deciding to shut his business down as this was not the first time he had been robbed. He had prayed for an answer. This owner truly felt God had sent us to pray for him. We gave him hope to continue.

The Greek Restaurant owner told us he feeds whoever comes into his restaurant. He located on Barton Street because he felt prompted to open his magnificent restaurant there. His restaurant truly was magnificent.

The co-owner of *Kenesky Sports & Cycle* commented, "These streets really need to be cleaned up. Do you think prayer will help?"

A Liquor store staff member commented after I explained why we were there, "You do know where you are, don't you?"

I explained, "Of course I do. We want to pray for the needs of your staff."

His eyes opened wide as he proclaimed, "What a great idea!"

The manager of *Hamilton Strip* exclaimed, "I never thought I would see the day someone would come in here and take a prayer request."

I explained, "We all have needs."

As I was leaving a flower shop located beside a spa, the store clerk warned, "You aren't going next door are you?"

"Of course, I am."

"No, you really don't want to go next door!"

"Yes, I really do want to go next door," I insisted.

At *Signature Spa* several women were standing around the front counter and a rather large gentleman sat behind a desk off to the side. I presented my spiel to the bouncer-sized fellow at the desk, ending with, "And, I think you need prayer for those eyes."

He explained that wallboard dust had gotten into his eyes while doing renovations. The doctor had given him several different medications, but nothing helped.

"We'll be praying for you." I assured.

When I joined the team on the sidewalk, we immediately prayed for his healing.

In three afternoons we completed our first entire route. So, on our fourth time out, about a month into this venture, we began our second trip down Barton Street. I had my cell phone, pen, paper, copies of another letter for each business, and this time, I felt to bring some money with me. I had never brought money with me before; I had never seen a reason to take money. About two blocks from our starting point, Don and I came to an abandoned building. At one time, this building must have been a banquet hall. Six wide steps lead up to the front door, but a thick iron chain hung from handrail to handrail across the bottom step to prevent the public from wandering up to the door. A gentleman, a street person, obviously undeterred by the chain, was sitting on the top landing. His back rested on the glass door—his belongings in bags on either side of him.

"I think we need to find out if this guy is okay," I said to Don.

Our street person was a soft-spoken man, aged beyond his years. The elements had definitely toughened his skin. A little into our conversation, I asked, "When is the last time you've eaten?"

Well, he couldn't really remember. He didn't ask for money or any kind of hand-out.

"Would you like something to eat?" I asked.

His eyes reflected great appreciation at the offer. Thinking of the fast food place a few buildings down, I suggested a few meal options, giving him a choice. He chose milk over pop. It was important for him to have milk and to look after his body. "Are you Christians?" he asked.

I cringed. I seriously do not like to be defined by that word. So many people are turned off by so-called Christians. "We are followers of Christ just trying to do our best," I qualified.

Don stayed with him chatting while I went to get the food. When I came back with his food he was very appreciative. He had been chatting with Don about *Mission Services*, but he wasn't sure where it was. We gave him directions, bus fare and a prayer. That was the only day I felt prompted to take money and that was the only day in a year and a half we ever came across a street person.

On our second time into the *Prince Edward Tavern*, the owner asked to speak to me in private. She had read the letter we had given her on our first visit. She wondered if I knew anyone looking for a job. She felt if we recommended a person that she would be able to trust this person not to steal from her. What an opportunity! Think about this. What is the likelihood that a regular at a tavern would be attending your church? Church-goers have to be willing to meet people outside the walls of the church if they want to be a positive influence.

A word of encouragement from a bartender could mean everything to someone who just lost his job and wants to drown his sorrows in a drink or seven. What would a kind word do for a lonely regular with no family? Let's drop the "holier than thou" attitude and go where we can meet lonely, hurting people. The owner of the *Prince Edward Tavern* opened my eyes to a need. Eventually I was able to refer someone for the job. Without a doubt, she became a comforting ear to a number of regulars.

Down the street at *Ever Convenience* the owner reported no problems since our last visit. He believed this was because of the prayers. The store had not been robbed and the owner noticed a more positive respectful attitude among many of the regular young people.

At the massage parlour the gentleman with the eye problem wasn't in. One of the ladies excitedly reported that he no longer had an eye problem. Two days after my last visit his eyes had been healed. This has been the topic of conversation in the place. She explained that he had been on many different types of medications and none of them had worked so they all knew it was the prayer. She confided that even he was admitting it might be the prayer.

By the time we finished a complete route from Gage to Locke we had visited 171 businesses. Our team completed the route three times each year for two years. Many of the business owners, managers and staff recognized our faces when we came through their doors.

Don and I were the regulars; others joined when they could. The store owners, managers and clerks were always friendly and appreciated knowing someone cared for them. Only once did a store employee laugh at us—only once in one thousand and twenty six visits. That ratio suggests people appreciate what the church has to offer, but on their turf.

On our visits we used commonsense and tried to be courteous at all times. We avoided causing embarrassment, never insisting on on-the-spot prayer. We avoided interrupting business or bothering customers. We were friendly and genuinely had nothing to gain. We simply promised to pray for needs, letting the people know someone cared, and in time we gained trust. Yes, in time, we built relationships. We didn't have a hidden agenda. We didn't gain trust and then ask for a donation. We simply cared.

Every visit to Barton Street became an amazing adventure. Three of these adventures stand out. By late summer of the first year, we had built a rapport with one of the co-owners of *Kenesky Sports & Cycle*. On this occasion, when we arrived the store was crowded. Hockey season was about to begin and many parents were having their children fitted for a new season.

My seventeen years as a hockey mom told me this was no time to distract staff. We certainly didn't want to interrupt business. I waved at the co-owner as I placed our letter on the front counter. He yelled across the store, "No, don't leave. Are you still praying for our business?"

"Yes," I responded.

"Well, I have a really bad back. Can you pray for me?"

Recognizing the store was crowded with customers, I replied, "Of course, I will add you to the list."

"No, I want you to pray for me right now."

That caught me by surprise; nevertheless I jumped into action. I put my hands on his back and prayed for him in his store in front of all his customers.

After we prayed, he proclaimed, "This feels better already."

One day before going out, we prayed specifically to meet with the owners and managers at every store. Marian was walking with me that day. You may recall, Marian was the one who had joined *Prayer at City Hall* because one night she had heard the repeated command, "Join the army at city hall."

On this particular day we were starting from the top of the route for the third time. Miraculously, at every store we were able to speak with the manager or owner just as requested in our prayer. At the Canadian Imperial Bank of Commerce (CIBC) when we asked for the manager, we were told she was not presently in the branch. We left our letter, started out the door, then practically bumped into the manager (who was wearing a name tag) on her way in. We introduced ourselves, pointed to the letter with the offer to pray for the people at the bank and then left marvelling at God's attention to detail.

At a department store, when we asked to speak to the manager he came out of his office, to meet us. I introduced myself, gave him the spiel and asked if there was anything we could pray about.

"Yes," he nodded. "I am addicted to pharmaceuticals and they are killing me. I don't want to be addicted. I've been addicted for a very long time. Please pray for me."

He gave us his name and we promised him we would be praying for him. We had never met the man before he shared his need. That took guts and trust on his part.

There were several massage parlours on Barton Street. On one of our visits to one of the massage parlours a large, well-endowed, scantily dressed, young lady was seated in a lounge chair. I introduced myself and asked if she had a prayer request. She gently looked at me as tears streamed down her face, "That is so nice. You really care about us don't you?"

She broke my heart as she continued to thank me. She took the letter asking if she could have a copy for herself.

Another time I found myself on the doorstep of yet another massage parlour. I waited in the front lobby until a young girl came out to greet me. She seemed very nervous and scared. I introduced myself, told her about our praying for businesses, and asked if she had a prayer request.

With fear in her voice she said, "Please don't ask me anything. This is my very first day."

I gave her the letter, and held her hand as she reached for it, "If you need anyone or anything you just call that number, okay?"

She took the letter. I could see she was afraid someone might be listening or watching her.

I left. As I walked across the street my heart ached. I kept thinking she couldn't be of legal age. *Where were her parents? Where was her mother? Why would she be in there?* I kept thinking about my own daughter, younger than this girl but likely not by much. *What would cause a young girl to take employment at a massage parlour? Why was I here today on her first day? Please, please Lord, tell me what to do.*

My mind was racing and my emotions were not in control, not good when I needed to use commonsense. Then I felt the prompt. *Of course...why didn't I think of that?* My cell phone held the number for the police department. I had a good reputation with the Chief of Police and his executive assistant. I could call them for advice. The Chief of Police wasn't in, but his executive assistant connected me to someone in vice. I explained the situation and within 45 minutes two vice officers were at that massage parlour. They asked the young lady to step outside, asked to see her identification and had a quiet conversation with her.

The police department called me later that day to let me know the girl was of legal age, though barely. The officers had had a positive talk with her and thought she wouldn't be working there any longer.

Was it a coincidence that on that day I walked that part of Barton Street? I don't believe there are any coincidences in life, but there are lots of adventures we don't see because we don't want to see them or can't be bothered to follow our promptings. I have no idea where that young girl is today, but in my heart I believe she understood on that day, that someone cared for her. Maybe when she felt no one else in the whole world cared for her, that day she felt someone cared.

People need to know that people care about them. As much as food and water, on the most basic level, people need to know someone cares. This can make a world of difference in their lives. Maybe, just maybe, the realization that someone cares can set them in a different direction on their life's journey.

The occult store, *6 Ways to Wisdom,* has been on Barton Street for many years. It was one of the stores I visited on our route. On one visit, after introducing our cause and handing the letter to the store clerk, I asked, "Do you have a prayer request?"

The clerk replied, "Yes, we could all use prayer." She gave me the name of the owner and her own name. I thanked her and let her know that we would be praying for the store, for the store owner and for her. I have come to realize that many people are searching to believe in something, someone, some higher power...a power outside themselves.

Now, if *the church* was doing a decent job conveying who Jesus Christ really is and what He has already done for each and every one of us, then maybe the *new age* population wouldn't be so large and growing larger. It is not anyone's job to pile shame, guilt and judgment on others. I love the story about Jesus and the so-called adulteress.

Jesus says to the crowd gathered to stone her, "You who have not sinned may throw the first stone." They all turned around and walked away because they all knew they had sin in their lives.

If you are talking to someone who doesn't attend church, ask them why they don't attend. One reason I hear over and over again, "Why would I go to church to be condemned and made to feel bad about myself by others in the church?"

Our job is simple; love others as we would like to be loved.

We can't make people change. Nobody changed me. Gentle promptings helped me change. These changes occurred gently and over time. Ultimately it was the Holy Spirit changing me, little by little, showing me the truth.

As church-goers, we shy away from getting to know *those* people, yet Jesus ate with *those people*. He ate with the tax collector. I am guessing, while He was eating with the tax collector, He was probably getting to know him and his family. I seriously doubt that Jesus was making the tax collector feel ashamed and guilty. I don't get the impression that Jesus was a Bible thumper. I do, however, know He shared stories, spent time with people, and was gentle and caring.

Sharon Boase, reporter for *The Hamilton Spectator,* got wind of the adventures happening on Barton Street and did an article. She was someone I could trust. Every time she wrote an article about an adventure she did it with care and respect. She always wrote accurately, truthfully and respectful of the people in her stories. I was so grateful for her skills.

For this story, Sharon interviewed store owners and took photos. Because of that article, the producer of *Listen Up TV* contacted me for an interview. From that interview others contacted me wanting information so they could begin a similar project.

I willingly shared our simple system and what we had gained through our experiences. To everyone who asked, I forwarded a copy of our letter. In sharing I always stressed the trust factor.

Those on Barton Street appreciated that we were a team of people from different churches and denominations. They appreciated that our churches had nothing to gain as we didn't belong to any of the churches on Barton Street. They mainly appreciated that we didn't have a hidden agenda. We truly just wanted to pray for their needs without judgment.

I knew when the time for walking Barton Street was ending. I was getting a prompting to run for mayor in the city of Hamilton in the 2006 municipal election. My commitments were shifting. Running for mayor was a big adventure, one that required a lot of preparation.

SEVEN

My Mom

Personally I find it easier to share my beliefs with someone I've just met, didn't know before, and likely will never meet again, than to talk about God with my extended family. Honestly, I was terrified when I felt this next prompting. I was terrified because the prompting had to do with my mom—not that my mom is difficult to get along with. On the contrary, she is very personable.

My mom was not a church-goer. She believed in God, but didn't talk to Him. I am sure at times she wondered if I had lost my mind and my senses. I had been told I was a little over the top. My extended family couldn't understand why I wanted to go to church for a morning service and then go for the evening service as well. They didn't understand each service was different.

Often my family would hold a family function on Sunday afternoon and inevitably this would last into the evening. I would need to choose between an evening service where I longed to be, and a family function which was also important to me. My family had a hard time believing I wasn't forced to go to church, that I actually enjoyed going.

My mom had retired and was living her dream. Everyone should live their dreams. My mom and her husband began by buying a former bed and breakfast in Port Dover. With major renovations, this old Victorian home with a big wraparound front porch and large front doors, became the fulfillment of my mom's dream: a bed-and-breakfast with full dining room facilities. The front doors lead into a large hallway with a beautiful wooden staircase up to second-floor bedrooms. My mom and her husband maintained a loft on the third floor as their own private quarters. There were a lot of stairs to climb in a typical day.

In July of 2003 my mom began experiencing extreme pain in one of her knees. For my mom to complain, the pain had to be excruciating. Being on her feet all day long and climbing those stairs didn't help matters.

She had seen her doctor, had tests and taken the prescribed pharmaceuticals. Nothing helped. The pain became so intense she preferred to sleep on a couch on the main floor to avoid the two flights of stairs to her bedroom.

Well, on the morning of July 23rd, I was having my usual early morning quiet time and once again I knew a prompting was coming. This time I was prompted to call my mom to tell her I would drive to Port Dover, lay hands on her knee and pray for healing.

My heart started to race. I was not doing this, no way. Oh, I wanted her to be healed, but what if I prayed for her and she wasn't healed? How would I ever explain that to her or anyone else in my family? If I prayed for her and she wasn't healed she would never believe me again. Worse yet, if she didn't get healed, this might totally turn her away from ever thinking about having a personal relationship with the Lord.

Inside I was freaking out. I was thinking about me—and justifiably so. My family wasn't exactly on board about my relationship with God. They labelled me "*whacko.*"

If God chose to heal my mom, she would be healed; but I had prayed with people in the past who were not healed. How could I explain that to my family? I had a hard enough time figuring it out for myself. So I wasn't expecting my mom to grasp the concept that some get healed and some don't. Basically my prompting translated into, "Hey Diane make a fool of your self. Let your family know you are truly loony."

Seriously, this was not an easy task to complete.

My mom struggled with understanding how God could allow someone like Paul Bernardo into heaven. According to scripture, if Paul Bernardo sincerely asked forgiveness for his grievous crimes he would be forgiven. If he then accepted Jesus as the one who paid for his atrocities, and he loved Jesus for it, the Bible says Paul Bernardo would go to heaven, and have eternal life. My mom felt that maybe she didn't want to go to the same place as a person like Paul Bernardo.

My mom is a good person. My mom has always helped people. So, she couldn't understand why she wouldn't just naturally go to heaven. The truth is we don't get to heaven by doing. So many people miss that point. It's all about our relationship with God.

To follow through with this prompting, I did some serious self-talk. Then I took a deep breath and dialled the number. Mom answered.

"Hi Mom, how are you doing? How is your knee?"

"Bad. Painful."

"Well mom, I was in prayer this morning and I feel I need to drive down there and put my hands on your knee and pray for you to be healed."

Silence!

Finally, she replied, "That's okay honey, you stay home. I don't need you to come here. I will be okay."

"Okay, bye."

Relief flowed through me. She didn't want me to come and pray for her. Great, fabulous, fantastic, what a relief—I wouldn't have to explain anything to her if she didn't get healed. *Well, Lord I did my part*. What a load off of my shoulders.

Normally my mom and I didn't call or see each other a lot. We were both extremely busy and I felt she had so much on her plate that when she had a day off (hardly ever) she deserved the time to herself. Two weeks went by and then she called me.

Mom got right to the point. "Hi Diane, how are you? You know when you last called me about coming to pray for me?"

"Yes," I said apprehensively, feeling a tightening in my stomach, as I prepared for her *are-you-crazy* speech.

"Well, I know you prayed for me when you hung up the phone. I needed to call you and tell you I've been healed ever since you called me that day to pray for me."

I was speechless.

She went on to say, "I haven't had a pain since you called. That's all I wanted to say, I should have called earlier but I was waiting to make sure it wasn't my imagination. I have to go now, bye."

I was stunned. I was excited, happy and grateful—but stunned. After our last conversation truly the only thing I remember is feeling relieved that she hadn't wanted me to come and pray for her. I know that I did pray for her, but I also know I was thinking more about myself after our conversation then I was thinking about her. That's the honest, human truth.

Sometime later, after my mom sold her bed-and-breakfast and had Sundays free, she and her husband began attending church—sporadically at first, but soon they became regular attendees. They began to enjoy the services.

Then in 2007 my mom and her husband began also attending small groups or evening services on Sunday. Yes, they went to church for morning service and then wanted to go back to attend an evening service. Oh, it gets better. I invited them to join us for a family dinner one Sunday evening. I was overjoyed to hear mom beg off, "I don't think so. We have small group on Sunday night and we don't want to miss it."

My mom and her husband had become *born-again* believers and were baptized. They had made the decision to invite Jesus into their lives. Being *born again* is an individual's decision. A baby doesn't inherit this new way of living from parents or receive it during a dedication, christening or baby baptism. New birth happens when an individual decides to put Jesus in charge of his or her life.

Developing this personal relationship with God is something that does not happen overnight. It's a relationship, a trust, an intimate knowing that takes time. God gently allows us to take our time. I love that. He has given us free will. He wants us not to feel obligated but to want to have a relationship with Him.

I absolutely know when you see a miracle you won't doubt His love, care, gentleness, guiding, prompting and kind desire for each and every one of us. He has no favourites and He desires each of us to have eternal life with Him.

EIGHT

Expecting the Unexpected

Our family is big on family gatherings and traditions. Throughout the year, four generations of family, including my three siblings, our parents, our children and grandchildren gather to celebrate birthdays, graduations and holidays—any excuse will do. Three times a year, Christmas, Easter and Thanksgiving, my aunt's family frequently join us. On these occasions we have a lot of people at the table.

My aunt and my mom are close; they went through their pregnancies together—need I say more? I am the oldest of the next generation, with a cousin a few months younger. My sister and brother have cousins their ages as well.

One of our favourite and most valued family traditions is our Thanksgiving Day gathering. Thanksgiving dinner is always celebrated on the Monday of the holiday weekend. We don't dress up for the occasion and we typically organize a potluck. We call it a potluck, but according to our tradition, we organize who is bringing what for the buffet. We traditionally eat at noon. No one goes hungry as we dig into the bountiful provision. When we have all eaten several helpings more than planned, there is barely room for dessert. That's okay, because traditionally we save our dessert for later after our traditional hayride. As my brother disappears down the road to borrow a tractor and hay wagon from his brother-in-law, the rest of us tidy-up, and organize blankets and chairs, and whatever else we need for the hayride. We all pile onto the wagon. A two-month-old baby holds the record for the youngest participating family member, and so far my grandmother in her late 70's holds the record for oldest. Thanksgiving usually involves great fall weather. Only once in my memory were blankets a priority. Once we had a light drizzle of misty rain, but not enough to get soaked. The last couple of Thanksgivings people have been in shorts.

For years now we have climbed aboard the hay wagon and putted over to Waterbrook Farm, on Springvale Road just outside Hagersville, where we ride horses. Waterbrook Farm was at the time a Christian children's summer camp. The campers at this 'farm camp' help out with chores such as feeding the animals and gathering eggs. Kids, especially kids from the city who haven't experienced farm living, love the atmosphere.

Our hayride on Thanksgiving Day 2005 started off like any other. When we turned into the lane at Waterbrook Farm, Matthew, the owner, welcomed us. As he loves to do, he showed the guys in the family his old motorcycle and other 'guy' stuff he had collected over the years. Then Matthew, my brother and a few others moseyed over to the tack shop to gather the saddles to saddle up the horses for our family's traditional afternoon ride.

The rest of us found other things to keep us busy. Some continued exploring through the 'guy' things in the covered utility shed. Some thought the buffaloes most interesting. Others, including myself, proceeded to the play area to watch over the younger children swinging and climbing. From there, we couldn't see the door of the tack shop or any of the saddling activity, and consequently didn't see the mishap.

We weren't even aware anything had happened until several of my nieces and nephews came running to the play area, "Aunt Diane, you have to come. Matthew fell!"

Why did they run to me? I worked in complimentary health and have an anatomy and physiology background, but what could I do?

Regardless, I went with them. As I rounded the corner of the tack shop, I saw Matthew lying flat on his back. My brother, who has first-aid training, was supporting one of Matthew's legs in a slightly elevated position. No one else was near. I kneeled at Matthew's head.

He had passed out and had just regained consciousness. As I knelt beside him, Matthew, who was obviously in severe pain, continued to move in and out of consciousness.

My brother commented, "I'm pretty sure the leg is broken. We called 911." I could see an ugly unnatural bulge under the skin at the ankle.

As Matthew came into consciousness once more, I leaned over him, "Matthew, are you listening to me? Stay with me Matthew. We are going to pray." By this time everyone had gathered around. To my left in my peripheral vision I could see my grown children. I could see others as well, but I wasn't focused on them. I was focused on Matthew.

I prayed. I can't remember what I prayed, but I prayed. I do remember feeling very different while I prayed. When I finished praying Matthew went out cold. The ambulance arrived. The two attendants efficiently splinted, padded and stabilized Matthew's leg. All the while, Matthew remained unconscious. One of the ambulance attendants privately told a family member that the leg was indeed broken and it looked like a bad break needing special attention.

They checked his pupil dilation, response, pulse—all the things they needed to check—then with help carefully loaded him onto the stretcher and drove off to the Hagersville hospital. Matthew's wife followed in her vehicle.

Matthew's family encouraged us to continue with our horseback-riding plans. It didn't take long to saddle the last few horses. We managed to enjoy our traditional ride along the lovely wooded trails.

After the ride, we helped unsaddle the horses and store the equipment. Then our family loaded back onto the hay wagon for the return trip to my brother's for our dessert smorgasbord. On the way, we chewed on soft pumpkin-shaped candies bought just for the occasion at the bulk food store. These candies have absolutely no nutritional value, but this is our tradition and we like our traditions.

Often my mom will bring crafts for the grandchildren to do when we return from the hayride. One year my mom brought several dozen pumpkins for us to decorate. She also brought paint so the smaller children could paint the pumpkins instead of using carving knives. She showed the rest of us how to carve pumpkins into vases. We cut an opening, dug out the pumpkin seeds and inserted dried grasses and flowers she had collected and brought with her that day. These became great outdoor decorations. Now you know why we don't get dressed up for Thanksgiving.

As all Thanksgivings must, the day came to an end. We had feasted, gone for our hayride, rode horses, and visited with family while doing a craft—pure, simple fun.

On this particular Thanksgiving Day I had driven to my brother and sister-in-law's on my own. On the way home, as I approached the town of Hagersville, I decided to detour to the hospital.

The emergency department at the hospital was one I had visited on several occasions when my children were growing up. The automatic doors at emergency slid open as I stepped into the front lobby. I looked right, then left, to see Matthew attached to an intravenous drip and lying on a stretcher in a smallish, well-lit room. His wife was sitting on a chair at his side. I introduced myself to her. She told me Matthew was and had been unconscious for some time; morphine does that. She pointed to the x-rays mounted in a light-box on the wall. We walked over to get a closer look, and she traced her finger along the obvious break. She explained that the doctor, certain this break would need special attention, had arranged for Matthew to see a surgeon the next day. This confirmed what the ambulance attendants had said about a bad break.

There wasn't much I could do. I simply said the obvious, "I'm sorry this happened. Is there anything I can get for you? Please give me a call if there is anything I can do." I wrote my telephone number on a piece of paper and gave it to her. Then I left.

Late Tuesday evening when I answered my office phone, I heard, "Hi Diane, this is Matthew." My brain was searching, *Matthew, Matthew, Matthew who?*

Matthew could sense I didn't know who he was and spared me embarrassment, "Matthew from yesterday, the broken leg." He caught me completely by surprise. I really didn't expect to hear from him.

"Matthew, how are you? Where are you calling from?" I asked. He explained that he was at home.

"I thought you were supposed to be in the hospital."

"So did I!" Matthew related his extraordinary story, "I was at Hagersville Hospital for a good while. They stabilized my leg, pumped me full of drugs, sent some drugs home with me and told me to go and see the surgeon today. My wife took me to the surgeon, he examined my leg and said it's not broken. He wrapped my leg, gave me some exercises to do and sent me home with drugs." Matthew continued, "My leg is still very sore. The muscles have all been stretched and bruised, but my leg isn't broken. I know it is a miracle."

"Diane," Matthew said, "I don't remember much, but I do remember you praying for me. I believe the Lord heard the prayers and He healed me." Matthew kept saying, "It is totally a miracle."

I was as amazed as Matthew. I believe that people can be healed, but I am always in awe when they are.

Over time I have been introduced to several members of Matthew's family—we happen to attend the same church. His family continues to talk about how Matthew was healed on that Thanksgiving Monday.

When Matthew called that Tuesday, it was later in the evening so I didn't have a chance to tell my family. The next morning I shared Matthew's telephone conversation with my daughter. This was the daughter who had attended the Toronto Airport Christian Fellowship with me. Very calmly in a *didn't-you-expect-that-to-happen?* tone, she said, "Well mom, you should have seen the way you prayed." She didn't say, 'Well mom, you should have *heard what you said* in that prayer.' No, she said, "Well mom, you should have seen *the way* you prayed."

"What do you mean?" I asked curiously.

"Well, the best way to describe it is there was power all around you. We could see it." Out of the mouths of babes! My daughter just expected Matthew to be healed. Oh, if only we could all have that degree of faith.

NINE

Hell's Angels

In the beginning my God adventures were launched with distinct promptings. I knew I had to do a memorial for Tim. Wray told me I had to go to the Toronto Airport Christian Fellowship. An inner voice assured me we were to buy the truck, just as I had to buy army boots, had to pray for Barton Street and was nudged to pray for my mom.

When I prayed for Matthew and when I came face to face with a Hell's Angel, I didn't need a prompting—I had come into a new awareness. I began to hear people's needs. I had come to a place where I could see the need in a particular situation and not be held back by fear. The Lord had freed me of the fear of what others would think, the fear of inadequacy, and the fear of failure. Through the promptings my faith grew. I realized I could only do what I could do and had to leave the rest to God. I had to trust God to do the rest in *His own time*. He knows what is best.

Be content but not satisfied has become my personal motto. Be content whatever the circumstance, but not satisfied to stay in one place for any length of time. If life is a journey then life is about moving, changing, going, growing, learning, and being curious and a little daring. When you travel or go on a journey there has to be a first time to a destination. Once you find a destination you like, you might return but there is always a first. So why is it so easy to travel to a new destination on a vacation, but often so extremely difficult to accommodate change in other areas of our lives?

One of the catalysts moving me along on my journey is my bucket list—things I want to do before kicking the bucket. For years I held the desire to own a motorcycle, a definite on my bucket list. I always loved riding on a motorcycle. When my husband and I met he had a motorcycle. He told me I was a good rider; I wasn't afraid to lean into the turn and I loved the feeling of the air and the sense of freedom. And, I knew how to change gears.

In the fall of 2000, I took a three-day motorcycle training course. After successfully completing the course, I could legally drive a motorcycle and had five years to acquire a full license. If I didn't complete the mandatory exit test within five years, I would have to start over.

I hadn't realized how fast five years can fly by. During those five years other matters had my attention. In my growing relationship with the Lord, I felt prompted to pursue my ordination. On August 20, 2004, I was officially ordained as a minister, under Gospel Crusade of Canada, now called Global Christian Ministry Forum, which meant I was legally recognized by the Province of Ontario to sign marriage licences. (My Biblical studies and ordination proved to be a good foundation for leading Prayer at City Hall.)

In the early spring of 2005, the Ministry of Transportation notified me by mail that in October 2005 my motorcycle license would expire. Had it been five years? I didn't have a motorcycle and hadn't ridden one since my course five years earlier on a borrowed bike. My husband hadn't owned a motorcycle for years. We simply weren't getting the use out of a motorcycle while the children were growing up and it seemed like a waste to have a bike sitting in the garage unused.

Whenever I talked about possibly purchasing another bike, my husband clearly indicated a lack of interest. He had owned a number of motorcycles since his youth and had outgrown the desire. He suggested I get my motorcycle since I had always wanted one, but he was sure he wasn't interested in riding anymore. What to do?

Finally in July, I called the Ministry of Transportation to find out about booking the motorcycle exit test. There were only a few openings available in my timeframe. What should I do? A motorcycle was a lot of money.

By 2005 I was back in top physical shape. My muscles had healed completely. For early- morning exercise, I would go to Princess Point in Hamilton and rollerblade along the picturesque bay front. As I skated along the rolling path lined with rocks and trees and water, I talked with God. On this particular day I said, "Lord, you know I would like a motorcycle. You even know my timeframe. If it's okay for me to buy a bike, please give me a sign. If it's not okay, I am good with that too."

Just before my first client arrived that day I had decided to book a motorcycle exit test. My reasoning was simple: if somehow I did get a bike, my test would be booked. If I didn't get a motorcycle I could cancel the exit test. This made sense to me.

Then, my first client arrived. I must have been oozing motorcycle. She looked around, "You know what…my husband has a Harley for sale. Would you be interested in it?" I couldn't believe my ears. *What did she just say?* For months I had been looking, considering the different brands and concluded if I was to get a motorcycle I would get a Harley.

She went on. "We just live around the corner if you are interested."

That was the sign I needed. She gave me her husband's work number. I called him as soon as she stepped out of the door. His motorcycle was the model I wanted, but the price was a little high. He had customized the Harley right out of my price range.

The next day I visited several Harley dealerships. The 2006 models were coming in the very next week so I was able to make a deal on a 2005 Red 883L Sportster. I was beside myself with excitement, like a satisfied kid on Christmas morning.

One Sunday in August on the way home from church, my husband said to me, "It's such a great day, I think I will take your bike for a ride."

Quickly I replied, "I don't think so. I'm going out on it this afternoon, and you need to buy your own bike."

So, he did. He reasoned he needed to buy a motorcycle if he wanted to spend time with me. Smart man I married.

Thus began our Friday the thirteenth adventure in Port Dover.

Every Friday the thirteenth motorcycle enthusiasts from across North America converge at Port Dover, Ontario. Port Dover is a small town nestled on the shores of Lake Erie, the home of the famous Arbor foot-long hotdog and trademark beverage, Golden Glow. *On the Fringe Custom Leathers*, a store geared to bikers, stocks up for Friday the thirteenth. Powell Park is packed with vendors of every description and music groups entertain from makeshift stages staggered along the main drag.

Friday the thirteenth not only attracts motorcycle enthusiasts like my husband and I, but it also attracts motorcycle gangs—the real gangs such as Hell's Angels, Satan's Choice, and the Red Devils. I am sure the event is a policing nightmare. The gangs have become quite the entrepreneurs. They set up tents where they sell t-shirts and other items with their gang colours.

What started in 1981 with a handful of friends wanting to get together has become a major event. Hard core enthusiasts show up whatever the month. During the warmer months motorcycles are parked on both sides of the street from the main corner in Port Dover out to further than the eye can see. On Friday the thirteenth in July 2007 when my husband and I rode into town with the Red Knights there was an added double row of motorcycles parked down the middle of the main street.

The Red Knights are an international motorcycle club for firefighters. I became an associate member after riding in a charity ride with the Red Knights out of Hamilton Chapter 14 while campaigning for mayor in the city of Hamilton. Whenever I have been out on a ride I am the only woman member rider (although there are spouses who ride as passengers with their Red Knight husbands). We always have a great time riding.

The Red Knights gathered at Rymal Road and Upper James in Hamilton that day as did many other clubs. We pulled out at 7:30 in the morning, thinking we had plenty of time to get good parking spots in Port Dover. Wrong. When we arrived an hour later, we had to park on the main drag; doubled up down the middle of the street, in the further-than-the-eye-could-see section. Actually we were so far outside town our bikes were the last allowed to park on the road. There was no walking back to the bikes for something in our saddlebags that day. Heavy motorcycle boots don't lend to walking distances and we did our fair share of walking just to get to the main activities.

I am not complaining. Friday the thirteenth in Port Dover is an awesome event. Even non-motorcycle enthusiasts can enjoy the activity, the sights, people-watching and, of course, the thong man. Every Friday the thirteenth the thong man dressed only in a thong rides into town and walks the streets. In the cooler months he wears his thong and chaps.

As we walked we were able to see every make, model, colour, customizing detail, and wild, wacky idea possible on a motorcycle. There was even a motorcycle customized with skeleton parts and a trailer shaped like a casket. Everyone should attend a Friday the thirteenth in Port Dover at least once in their life, just for the experience.

That July day we literally walked shoulder to shoulder shuffling along with thousands upon thousands of people. My crossing the street through the crowd to look at a white t-shirt hanging on display (anything but black) proved impossible.

Our Red Knights chapter broke up into smaller more manageable groups for taking in the sights. My husband, our friend Rick and I managed to stay together in the crowd. We walked from the very, very far end where our motorcycles were parked to the lakefront where the boats were docked and more venders pitched. As Harley riders, we were in search of the Harley tent to pick up our Friday the thirteenth pins.

Once that was accomplished, buying t-shirts to commemorate the day became the only remaining must. This was something the guys wanted to do. Personally, I didn't want another black t-shirt and have never wanted a t-shirt with skulls. Thus my choice was limited.

Pins and t-shirts in hand, we were on the look out for a place to sit, eat and get a cold beverage.

On our way back up the street towards our motorcycles we stopped at a beer garden. Inside this tented beer garden, with three helmets in hand, I bee-lined to an empty spot at a picnic table, while the guys split up to purchase food and cold beverages.

A picnic table never felt so good. I put our purchases in each of our helmets, placed the helmets on the table and waited. I was hungry and thirsty. My warm bottled water wasn't cutting it. Yes, I, an ordained minister, was looking forward to a cold glass of beer—everything in moderation. I normally don't like beer but every now and then it is refreshing.

In due time the fellows, food and drink in hand, squeezed in beside me. After we refreshed ourselves, several other Red Knights wandered into the beer garden and joined us. Rick and my husband stood. I was still sitting at the picnic table.

At this point, I wasn't focused on conversation as I needed to use the ladies room. Thankfully, the organizers of Friday the thirteenth always have plenty of portable facilities available just for women. Like most women, I never delight in using portable facilities, but as I was almost busting....

Returning to our picnic table, I noticed someone sitting in my spot—not just someone, but someone with gang colours. I could be sure the badges on his leather vest were not for helping little old ladies across the street. Those badges were likely for accomplishing some sort of activity worthy of jail time.

I stopped in my tracks, all of our stuff was right there on the table in front of him. I looked at him. He looked at me and asked, "Am I in your spot?"

Not batting an eye I replied, "If you move over a bit I can sit beside you." He wiggled to the right and I sat down.

As soon as I took my seat, he leaned toward me and said, "Aren't you afraid of me?" There was no mistaking that he was a member of the Hell's Angels out of Kitchener.

I leaned back toward him, "No, I am not afraid of you."

With the corner of my eye, I could see my husband and the rest of the guys talking and laughing. Later they told me they had heard the gang biker ask if I was afraid of him, and they had come to the unanimous conclusion, "Buddy, you should be afraid of her!" I took that as a compliment.

The biker confided, "Most people are afraid of me." I just shrugged my shoulders and gave him a look that said I didn't know how to answer. He continued, "I had to sit down: my back is killing me. I couldn't even ride my bike today. I had to come in the van with all the gear."

"Really, you have a sore back?" I questioned. "May I pray for you?"

"What?"

"May I pray for you? I am a minister and I believe in the power of prayer. I also believe that you sat here for a reason. Jesus wants to heal you. So may I pray for you?"

"Okay," he replied. The internal debate was written on his face. *Do I really want to have her pray for me? I would like to get rid of this pain, but…?*

"May I lay hands on you?"

He did a double take then looked me straight in the eye, "Whhhhhhaaaaattt!!!!!"

"It's the way I pray. I will just take my hand and lay it on your back and then pray for you."

He looked at me with one eye kind of squinted. "Okay," he said hesitantly.

I slid my hand under his leather vest, over his t-shirt in the area of his lower back.

"Why did you put your hand there? That is exactly where my back hurts."

I replied, "That's where I felt to lay my hand; the Holy Spirit is guiding me."

He just looked at me.

Now, I wouldn't do the prayer justice if I tried to repeat it here. Usually when I am spirit-led in a prayer, I don't remember what I pray. I do know I prayed for healing.

"Thank you. That's the nicest f*%king thing anyone has ever done for me."

"You are welcome," I said.

"You know, I was raised in a home where my parents went to church, but they sure didn't show us what they talked about in church," he related. "So you are a minister? Like the kind that can marry people?"

"Yes, and bury people," I answered. "That's the part that is really hard for me. When I do a funeral service and I don't know where the person is going. I know they are going somewhere but where the somewhere is I am not always sure. They are either going to heaven or they are going to hell. To me going to heaven is a lot easier and nicer then going to hell for eternity, and most people don't know that God desires everyone to go to heaven and it begins with having a personal relationship with Jesus. He forgives everyone if they ask. Can you imagine all they have to do is ask?"

He just looked at me, "You really believe this shit don't you?"

"Yes I do, with all my heart. You know why I can believe it?"

"Why?"

"Because I have witnessed it personally in my life," I explained. "I have been physically and emotionally healed. I really believe we were meant to meet here today. You do understand that when you are healed, it has nothing to do with me? It's all about Jesus."

"Okay."

I am sure he didn't totally understand, but I wanted to make it clear that I didn't hold any power and the healing didn't come from me.

The biker went on to tell me more about his family and the confusion of religion. I explained that I don't like religion and rules either—that in my opinion Jesus Christ isn't about rules. I also mentioned that I was ordained under Gospel Crusade which is non-denominational, which means we believe in the whole gospel including the parts about healing.

As our conversation continued other members of his gang gathered in the beer garden. One member came over to him and motioned him to join the rest of them, which he did. He thanked me as he left to join his group.

My husband, Rick and I stayed another 20 minutes before we decided it was time to continue up the street to our motorcycles.

As we were leaving, the biker eyed me from where he stood with his gang. He was on the far side of the circle. I reached across the group and shook his hand, "It was really nice to meet you. Don't forget what I told you." As we continued on our way out, I could hear the other members questioning him about me. Without any embarrassment or hesitation, he boldly declared, "She prayed for me and believes my back will be healed."

I did my part; I was leaving the rest up to God, as we should.

Don't tell me being a Christian is boring—I know otherwise. I left that beer garden so high on life I could have flown home.

The following year as I prepared for the next warm summer Friday the thirteenth, I mentioned to a friend whom I had previously told this adventure, "I wonder if I will run into that biker again."

To which she responded, "Why would you even think he would still be in that gang?"

Good question.

TEN

The Phoenix Rising Center

I have a dream—an enormous dream. This dream is much bigger than I, so big only God can make it happen. My dream is called the Phoenix Rising Center. With all my heart and soul I know this vision will come to be.

I didn't come up with the name—I would have chosen a less controversial name. Good *Christians* have told me repeatedly that the name Phoenix Rising sounds *new age*. According to the dictionary the phoenix is a bird in Egyptian mythology. This bird lived in the desert for five hundred years and then consumed itself by fire, later to rise from its ashes, renewed with amazingly beautiful red and purple feathers.

Phoenix Rising is a perfect name for the center as envisioned. It will be a place where people will be welcome regardless of financial status, culture, or religion. Everyone will be accepted, simply because Jesus never turned anyone away. That love, the love one will feel while at the center is bound to consume each one like a consuming fire and each will rise renewed. The Phoenix Rising Center is all about the love of Jesus.

People shouldn't be dying because they can't afford natural procedures not covered by our Ontario Health Insurance Plan (OHIP). As an iridologist, someone who works with people in a holistic approach to wellness, it's frustrating when patients are not able to take full advantage of my skills and experience because they don't have the money. I have seen people— especially women—deny themselves their health because they feel the family can't afford nutritional supplements or better food choices.

At the Phoenix Rising Center people with all types of physical dis-ease will be able to come and be seen by practitioners in both the holistic and medical fields—practitioners not competing with one another, but combining efforts for the person's best interest. We will have a facility where patients can be monitored while fasting or receiving care. We will also have a retreat center where people can attend workshops or spend needed time alone. A team will work to create a wellness plan for each individual.

This dream for the Phoenix Rising Center began to take shape in 2002. One Tuesday in October of that year an acquaintance came to me with a business card. "You are going to need a lawyer. Here is the name of a lawyer," she said.

"Why would I need a lawyer?"

She shrugged her shoulders and handed me his card. That night I had the dream. Now I have had dreams before, but this dream was very different—it came as a message, a prompting.

In my spirit I knew I should pay special attention. The dream was about a healing center, and held a warning. "Beware, people will try to hold you back, family, friends and… (I am not willing to share this particular part just yet). You need to walk on, *be bold*."

I awoke and sat right up. The feeling to pay attention was still strong. I couldn't go back to sleep. So, very early Wednesday morning I went downstairs to my quiet place. I grabbed a blanket, wrapped myself up and sat on my big pillow on the floor. I pulled out my journal, my Bible, pen and highlighter as I always do when I come to this corner of the front room to have a conversation with my Heavenly Father.

I prayed, "Lord if You want a healing center, You need to show me the way. What do You want it to be called?" Before I could finish the question, the words came: *Phoenix Rising*.

"What?" I responded.

Then I audibly heard, "Phoenix Rising."

Then I saw a vision of what the Phoenix Rising Center will look like. I saw a lot of land somewhere in the country, but not in the boondocks. The place is accessible, driver friendly, within an hour or so of an airport. There are three large facilities on the land. The buildings are scattered with the retreat center furthest from the road. There are acres of naturally landscaped space between the buildings. I also saw a body of water, a pond or something, where people could walk and sit.

The clinic is four stories high. An extraordinarily welcoming entrance greets everyone coming in through the main doors. All the assessment rooms are on the main floor. Here is where qualified, certified and accredited natural practitioners, as well as medical doctors who believe in combining medicine with a natural approach to wellness, assess patients. Gathering rooms where the wellness team gathers to come up with a plan of care for each person are also on the first floor.

Treatment rooms are on the second floor. People who needed to stay overnight or longer for their ongoing care, stay on the third floor. When a person arrives at the Phoenix Rising Center they are immediately assessed and their wellness plan is established. Patients will get answers as soon as possible—no waiting six weeks for results, and another four weeks to see the specialist.

In my personal experience the waiting and wondering was the hardest. I agree with the proverb, "Where there is no vision, the people perish." When we have an answer, we at least know what we are dealing with and can start to explore options.

I truly hope we don't need a whole floor for administration, but administration will be on the fourth floor of the clinic. This makes good sense. Why put healthy administrators on the first floor, while people who are sick travel the distance to other floors?

The overall focus of the clinic is to discover the root cause of a person's health challenge—not just to treat symptoms. Although the clinic is for all dis-ease, I know the center will specialize in helping people who have been diagnosed with cancer.

Of course there is a cafeteria. The cafeteria will follow a healthy nutritional program—not Canada's food guide.

I envision the retreat center as a critical part of an entire wellness complex. Natural and medical care will be available on site at the retreat center for those who require monitoring during extensive fasting and for juicing. Research has proven that emotional issues can create physical issues in the body. These emotional issues manifest in specific organs. Specialists who understand this concept can trace out a person's emotional issues. From a practitioner's point of view, pinpointing the emotional challenge is the easy part. Helping the person to understand and deal with the issue is the real challenge. What took years to manifest and create dis-ease in the body is not about to give up the fight and leave the body without a battle. The war is won here. Therefore, a wellness center needs a retreat center.

The retreat center looks and feels like a comfortable cozy cottage in a country setting. People can go for walks, or just sit surrounded by God's beauty. The retreat center has trained counsellors who are led by the Holy Spirit with a gift for listening for emotional needs. The retreat center is a place where people can come for physical, emotional and spiritual restoration and will accommodate people who come for retreats or healing conferences of varying lengths from one to seven days.

We humans are three parts: body, soul and spirit. Our soul involves the mind, will and emotions and needs to be filled up on a regular basis. Many people ignore their spirit and their soul. They don't know why they were created and who they truly are. When people don't have focus, they lose purpose and meaning. Every day is just another day and they aren't sure why they are living. *Where there is no vision the people perish.*

The auditorium will have a minimum capacity of 2000 with elevated seating for ultimate viewing. It will house state-of-the-art sound and audiovisual systems. This is a place to educate and train.

It is possible to guide a person to total wellness but in most cases people will slowly move back to old habits if they do not have reinforcement. This support system involves suitable training and education about new living habits. We all need a support system for consistent renewing and refreshing. In the auditorium speakers will teach, train and inspire listeners to continue their journey in total wellness so they will be able to "live on go."

Worship bands will also have a part. Music and worship is soothing and refreshing. Imagine 2000 people worshipping and praising God's name, raising their hands or quietly taking in the loving feeling. The auditorium is as essential as the other two buildings.

That is my vision. That Wednesday morning in October 2002 I wrote and drew pictures, words, phrases and feeling as they came to me. I have rewritten my journal notes here. I know this is not about me. It is so big I could never do this on my own, nor would I try.

The Phoenix Rising Center is built on what Jesus has commanded us to do—love. The greatest gift one could ever give to another is love. People can choose to take advantage of the retreat center and auditorium at their own discretion; these services aren't mandatory for receiving care at the clinic. Seminars, speakers and their topics will be announced beforehand and anyone can choose to attend or not.

These things will be offered because they are beneficial. Personally I believe Jesus Christ is the Saviour. I believe He was born of a virgin, was crucified, rose three days later and I believe in eternal life. I believe there is heaven and hell and I choose heaven. That's my talk. Jesus walked *His* talk. If I follow Him, I must walk mine. He will do His part in His own timing as I do my part.

On Thursday, the day after writing down all these things, I felt prompted to contact the lawyer on that business card my acquaintance had given me. I explained my need for charitable status. With charitable status the center would be able to accept donations. He wanted to know a little about the project. I explained briefly with as much detail as necessary to understand the concept. He kept saying, "You really need to move on this." As our conversation ended, he promised to fax me the required paperwork.

In my view, incorporation and charitable non-profit status are important for the Phoenix Rising Center to sustain itself. When I was sick back in 1995 my husband's benefits would cover pharmaceutical prescriptions, but nothing with a holistic natural approach. We only had to pay fifty cents per prescription. I got so desperate I eventually tried some of the prescribed anti-depressants, painkillers and anti-inflammatory pills. They made me feel worse. I not only still hurt all over but felt groggy, stupid and disoriented as well. I was in a daze even after trying different dosages.

I know in my own life and in my dis-ease, no prescription drugs would have helped. They would have masked the symptoms and never reached the root cause of my health challenges. I remember the sacrifices we had to make as a family because I wasn't working and was spending considerable funds on natural supplements and organic foods.

There are many people who truly can barely feed their family, let alone spend extra on proper nutritional supplements or fresh fruits and vegetable on a daily basis. Here in Canada, in Ontario, in the Hamilton Golden Horseshoe 100,000 children live in poverty—that's only the children.

Most people with dis-ease can't work or shouldn't be working. They should be resting. They shouldn't have to worry about how they are going to pay for their wellness care. The Phoenix Rising Center will be a place where all people, no matter what their financial situation, will have a personal plan of care and a choice for total wellness. Thanks to the non-profit charitable status this wellness will not have a price tag.

The funding for the center will come through donations. I believe funding will come flooding in because people will be healed. Families won't lose their mothers, or sisters, or daughters, or brothers, uncles, fathers or grandparents because they didn't have the money. Those who have more will give more. Those who have little will give as they can and it will mean as much as those who have more. Also, fundraising events will subsidize the center. Every donation will receive a charitable tax receipt. I believe this is the vision God gave me for the center.

Early Friday morning of the week of my vision, my fax machine spit out the lawyer's paperwork. It read, "In order to proceed you need to submit the following information with a cheque for five hundred dollars." My stomach went into a knot. I did not have five hundred dollars. I did the only thing I knew to do; I literally lifted the paperwork to the heavens and prayed, "Lord if you want this center, if You want me to continue with this charitable donation registration, then You Lord are going to have to make this happen." I put the paperwork on my desk, went back upstairs and continued to prepare for my workday, which was scheduled to be a very full day.

I didn't tell anyone about the fax or its contents. In fact I hadn't yet mentioned my vision to anyone. Then just before my first client arrived, my phone rang. Deb, one of my patients, explained she needed to see me right away.

I didn't have time for her. "Deb, I have a really tight schedule today. I am not sure when I am even going to eat lunch. Can I book you in next week?"

"No I have to see you today. I only need five minutes, seriously that is all I need is five minutes," she insisted.

I could hear the desperation in her voice, although I couldn't understand her dire need. I always leave a window of about fifteen minutes between patients to allow for extra concerns and paperwork. I don't like to keep patients waiting and I like to give my patients a feeling of confidentiality especially if one is leaving my office after a tearful emotional release, which is very common—I should have bought shares in Kleenex. Many times I have dealt with clients whose physical dis-ease has manifested from emotional issues. Our bodies are so amazing! They give us signals telling us something is wrong, although we seldom listen. The biggest or most harmful challenge to the body is the *secrets* we keep hidden inside.

Deb arrived right on time. I was leaning back on the front of my desk eating an apple when she walked into my office. Deb was serious and sombre; I could tell she had been crying. "What's wrong?" I asked.

As tears welled up in her eyes, she explained, "I want you to understand there are no strings attached. I felt the Lord telling me this morning to bring this to you." She handed me a white legal-size sealed envelope. She composed herself somewhat and continued, "Diane I have never done this before. I know it is a step of obedience for me....You use this for whatever you want. Get your book professionally edited or pay for a professional team to do a video of you speaking—whatever you want." (At the time I had just completed a draft for another book called *I'm Frustrated*.)

I knew immediately how I would use the money. I handed her the fax from the lawyer. I also told her how I had raised the fax to God and prayed. I hadn't opened the sealed white envelope so I had no idea what it held, but I didn't even need to open it. As Deb read the fax she burst into tears and confirmed that she had put five hundred dollars in the envelope.

I spent that evening completing the lawyer's paperwork and sent it with a cheque for five hundred dollars by express post the next day to apply for the incorporation and charitable registration. We still needed to come up with another three hundred dollars but I was convinced that would not be an issue nor was it. The final three hundred dollars came in the same way as the first five hundred dollars.

To proceed with the charitable registration status I needed a board. Deb became my very first board member.

Apparently some people wait months upon months and even years to receive their incorporation papers and then their charitable registration status. Some organizations never qualify for their charitable registration status and are denied. In May of 2003, seven months after the dream, a large brown envelope addressed to the Phoenix Rising Center arrived.

I carefully, excitedly opened the envelope. The Phoenix Rising Center had obtained its charitable organization number on March 3, 2003. For me, this was significant. In late 2002 and into early 2003 I had heard repeatedly, from different Christian groups, about the significance of 03-03-03—anything done on that day would be greatly blessed by God. Whatever was done, or begun on that day would be special. Even though it was not highlighted, underlined or in any way distinct from the rest of the print on that document, the date jumped out at me.

I envisioned once the center became incorporated and had its charitable status, everything would just happen. And why shouldn't I think that? The five hundred dollars came just like that, the following three hundred dollars came just like that. I had a board in place, so let the rest of the stuff happen.

Well, nothing happened except the original board, changed. One of the original board members passed away, another moved away and yet another felt his involvement would conflict with another project which might be able to provide funding to the center. Over time three new members came onboard.

The secretary of the Phoenix Rising Center board and I worked with an organization that specialized in matching people who wanted to be on a board with boards. Nothing, absolutely nothing came from all that work. Believe me, a lot of time and effort had been put into "trying to make things happen."

We acquired a website. A professional fundraiser worked free for almost a year with the understanding that when we were ready to begin building he would have the opportunity to apply to head the fundraising. Apparently as professional fundraising goes; it's a feather in a cap to be the fundraiser for a new building project. Through his efforts two donations totalling less than a thousand dollars came in. A lot of effort was put forth on both our parts with little to show for it.

What was going on? I realized what I was doing wasn't working. Maybe I wasn't supposed to do anything yet. So in my prayers for the Phoenix Rising Center, I said, "Lord I will be your mouthpiece and I will leave the rest up to you." I now had to stand by my words; I had to walk my talk.

I truly believe people are ready for a different approach to disease. In 1931 Dr. Otto Warburg won the Noble Peace Prize for medicine. He said, "*Cancer, above all other diseases, has countless secondary causes. But, even for cancer, there is only one prime cause. The prime cause of cancer is the replacement of the respiration of oxygen in normal body cells by a fermentation of sugar.*"

The body has the ability to heal itself. Our body automatically repairs and replaces cells on a daily basis. We need to understand how to help our bodies by removing toxins and introducing nutrients. I believe we can also help the body by removing fear—the fear of cancer. Many people think about cancer as soon as they realize something is wrong with them. I believe dwelling on the fear is very counter-productive and causes further disease.

We are ready for a different approach to health and wellness in this country. I believe the land, or money to buy the land for the Phoenix Rising Center, will be donated. When the time is right, it will happen. The first eight hundred dollars was provided when it was needed, and the rest will be provided as well.

It's not easy waiting, but I believe lives will be saved—and like the phoenix—consumed and born again.

ELEVEN

The Best is Yet to Come

Worse than being blind would be to be able to see but not have any vision — Helen Keller

Many people don't understand why I choose to follow promptings. Some people have told me how stupid I look believing what I believe. Last Christmas we were at a friend's home for a get-together when someone confronted me, "You don't really believe that stuff do you, that God stuff?"

"Of course I do," I responded.

I wasn't the one who brought up the subject; I wasn't even talking about God. Why do people routinely challenge me about God? Could it be they are curious? Could it be they are ready to hear about God? Could it be they are tired of feeling they have to do everything on their own? Could it be people are searching and need to talk to someone? If Christians stay within the four walls of their church buildings who will talk with these people? Church has to fulfill the needs of people and therefore go to where people are. A church building is a place for people to get filled and then go out into the world—workplace, neighbourhood, schools, anywhere and everywhere every day.

Some think being a Christian is boring and restricting. Well, my life is anything but boring. Who would have thought Diane Marie McLaughlin, conceived in lust, abandoned by two earthly fathers, and abused at a young age, would grow up to be Diane Marie Elms, who can pick up the phone and have a conversation with the Chief of Police of a city of over a half million people, run for mayor, pray face to face with those in authority, lead citywide events, pray for people and see them healed, be on television and speak in front of thousands (I'm not done but the sentence is getting too long). There are newspaper articles about my adventures that have reached international audiences, encouraging others to do what I did.

Some say being a Christian means you have to be weak and take crap. Some may look at the story of Jesus' life and think he was weak and took crap from those in earthly authority when he didn't defend himself, but He wasn't weak. He cleared a church of marketplace vendors by overturning tables and demanding they get out, that they stop making a house of worship into a den of thieves. There is nothing weak about walking out, or following through with a prompting. This takes strength and stamina. Being a Christian means paying the difference when a sales clerk undercharges. It means not screaming with road rage and issuing the three-finger salute (while mindlessly proclaiming your love for Jesus on your bumper) as you pass what you judge to be an idiotic driver. Actually it means not judging people at all. It means holding your tongue, not blowing up, not telling someone you think they are a good for nothing $#*&%)(*%.

A Christian learns to hold their tongue which, for some of us, takes more strength than letting the tongue flap. A Christian gives back the fifty cents or eight dollars or eight hundred dollars if a mistake has been made. What takes more strength, courage and character, keeping the money, or giving it back?

We all make mistakes. Mistakes are only a negative if you don't learn from them; I've made a lot of mistakes in my life. A lot of my mistakes were made when I was angry, frustrated or felt like I had to do everything on my own. During those times, I would have loved to have someone else help me or guide me, but I felt alone—me against the world. I bought into that perverted concept of life.

Now I am grateful to know I am not alone and never was, even when I thought otherwise.

I discovered some truths. One of these truths is that I am created in God's image. We all are. Not only are we created in His image, but He is also our Creator. Most creators of anything—a work of art, music, whatever—want the best for their creation. God wants the very best for us. Since I am convinced He only wants the best for me, I have to trust He will guide me, if I let him. How does He guide me? He does this through promptings, scripture, prayer, and wise counsel. I realize prompting is only one of the ways He guides me.

He prompts, but He also allows freewill. I wouldn't want a forced friendship. And, I wouldn't want my children to fear me or jump when I walk into a room. I want to have a relationship with them. I want to have conversations with them. I want them to appreciate me because they respect me not because I command it. I want my children to know I care about them and only want the best for them. I want them to trust me. I want my children to grow and become all they were meant to be. I see their potential. I want to encourage them and cheer them on. I want for my children what

God wants for His children, for me and you. So, if He wants the best for me and He knows my full potential, then it makes sense to listen to His guidance, and to follow His promptings.

If He hadn't prompted me to pray for Stelco, I still might not be praying in public. Think of all the adventures I would have missed. If He had not prompted me to go to the Toronto Airport Christian Fellowship I might be in a wheelchair today, instead of being a vibrant, energetic, healthy person who rides a motorcycle. If I had not followed the first prompting, if I had been too afraid or weak to trust or unwilling to dig deep within, I probably wouldn't be writing this book today.

With each prompting, I grew. He knows my full potential. I don't. I want Him to keep guiding me to be all that I can. I don't want to miss any of His adventures. I truly believe the best is yet to come.

When I became sick in 1995 I would have described myself as a positive person, and for the most part I was, but there was a part of me that worried. That part had to be dealt with. My physical healing included an emotional healing. I didn't understand the negative hold my emotional state had on me. I thought I had it all together or at least more together than most. I seriously hadn't recognized my pitiful emotional condition. To help the healing process, I read, took courses and even trained as a counsellor.

My healing process will be a big part of my next book. It is important for people to know what is happening inside: thoughts are powerful. Even the traditional medical field is admitting thoughts and emotion play a big part in physical health.

During my healing process, I realized that like an athlete, I needed a coach. I needed someone to tell me I am loved, I am good, I am accepted, I am beautiful, I have potential, I am smart and I am wanted. I needed someone to tell me these things on a daily basis until I could believe them when others were telling me differently. Most people won't tell you *in words straight out* that you are ugly, nobody wants you and nobody cares about you. They tell you by their *actions*. If they say one thing yet do another, it becomes confusing, especially for a little girl. That little girl grows up with confusion inside, confusion poking its ugly head into everyday life causing more confusion. The cycle doesn't end until deep inside the big girl knows the truth.

I chose God in all three persons to be my personal coach, to encourage me and guide me to my full potential. He is the only one who knows my full potential. It only makes sense to listen to Him. The ignorant don't know they are ignorant. People can't know they are lacking information they don't even know about.

In the introduction I mentioned that my biological father walked out of my life when I was a toddler. When I found out that the man I called my father wasn't my biological father, I started to look for my birth father. I didn't have much to go on. Periodically I would do an internet search. Then when I was around forty-four, I found him. I let my husband call the telephone number I had been given. I didn't want to create a challenge in this man's home by having a woman asking for him. My husband told him who I was and that it would be up to him to contact me if he chose.

Within minutes he called back. For the next eight years he would call me regularly. He sent flowers to me for every occasion and sometimes for no occasion. Once, he even flew to Toronto and met my husband and me for lunch.

But, he never told his family about me. He never signed any of the cards or notes on the flowers. I never called him—my choice, because from the beginning I made clear I wouldn't be part of a lie. If he wanted to contact me that was his choice, but until he told his family about me, I wouldn't contact him. After eight years I drew the line. I realized we had developed an unhealthy relationship. It felt oddly like being part of an illicit affair. My family knew my situation, but my biological father was telling his family lies, always contacting me secretly. I gave him the ultimatum: either tell your family or don't contact me again. He hasn't contacted me since. His actions speak louder than his words. He said, "I want you to know I love you. I never forgot about you. I thought about you all the time." Yet his actions prove otherwise.

From personal experience and through working with clients, I know many people have a difficult time relating to a loving heavenly Father, when their earthly parents are or were unloving.

I am not blaming parents for every mixed-up confused person. Parenting is not easy and we are bound to fail somewhere. I have yet to meet a person born with a manual attached. My three children are each different. Just when I figured I knew a few things, my next, totally different child was born—and back to the drawing board. Wrap those issues up with my hang-ups, and errors are bound to happen.

Parents will fail more than once. Some parents will fail miserably. If your parents failed miserably, you will have trouble calling God, "Father." You will have no basis for understanding a parent's love; or else maybe you'll understand a parent's love as something you want to run from. We need to deal with all that junk stuck inside.

I needed help. It took me a long time to trust enough in order to say, "Heavenly Father." When I said it—or rather, wrote it in my journal for the first time—I realized immediately what I had done and it felt so good. That feeling definitely had been missing in my life.

I was the first one in my family to be baptised. I was christened or dedicated as a child but actual full-immersion baptism and being *born again* were decisions I had to make for myself. I chose to go into that tank of water and confess in front of people, "Jesus is my personal Saviour." I chose to make Him the Lord of my life. The whole experience can be compared to the phoenix rising from the ashes to be born anew, a beautiful bird with red and purple feathers.

My family had a hard time handling the transition to my new life. Some people are fortunate to be born into a Christian family. They grow up believing and following Jesus. My immediate family all had to adjust when I decided to follow promptings and have God be my coach.

My family has admitted I have embarrassed them. More than once as we left the house, my daughter would beg, "Can today just be normal?" What is normal? I expect great things to happen on a regular basis.

Just a few days ago I was driving down a middle lane of Hamilton's multi-lane one-way Main Street, when I noticed a street person sifting through a garbage container on the sidewalk. In my heart I wanted to stop and give her some money. She was bundled up, the hood of her bulky dark jacket pulled tight around her face. She wore blue jeans and work boots and was pulling one of those upright, rectangular, two-wheeled bundle buggies. The buggy was overflowing with earthly possessions wrapped in tattered green garbage bags. People were waiting for the bus beside the garbage she was working on, but she didn't panhandle. She didn't bother the people. I'm not sure if she saw them or if they noticed her. But I noticed her. I kept saying, "Okay Lord, clear the traffic. I need to get over two lanes and park."

Traffic cleared and I was able to make a left onto Dundurn Street and pull into the plaza parking lot. I parked, grabbed some money from my wallet—not a lot but enough to buy a few meals—waited for the traffic light to change, and walked across the street where we met at the corner. She was making her way from garbage container to garbage container pulling her possessions along with her.

She was probably about 25 years old, but life on the streets had aged her considerably. She was clean, much cleaner than many street people; she walked with her head down not looking at anyone. I tapped her shoulder. She slowly turned towards me and lifted her head. Her eyes spoke of sadness. I took her hand, turned it over and put the money in her palm. I closed her fingers around the money. She looked at me and asked, "What is that for?"

"Just because," I said, then headed back to my orange Avalanche. I didn't tell her about God. I didn't pray with her. I didn't, because I wasn't prompted to do those things. My part was to give her the money. As I waited at the corner for the traffic light to change, I heard her voice but didn't catch her words. I turned and looked at her. She smiled and said, "Thank you." I smiled back and waved goodbye.

She had smiled a smile that said, "Thank you for making me feel special." If I had gone with my own agenda, Bible thumping perhaps, that would have taken away from what was accomplished. My role was simply to let her know someone cared. It might take the next person or the next person or maybe the twentieth person telling her she is special before she will be ready to hear about Jesus.

There are many adventures and promptings that I haven't shared in this book. The majority of my promptings are extremely personal, just for me. Some promptings I haven't made sense of yet. I know there are many more promptings and adventures to come. This journey doesn't end until my time on earth is finished.

Some of us are blind to promptings and some of us refuse to acknowledge promptings, but I believe we all receive them. I hope reading my adventures will help you choose to trust your promptings.

In the introduction to this book, I referred to John 10:10 in the Amplified Bible, ***"The thief comes only in order to steal and kill and destroy. I came that they may have and enjoy life, and have it in abundance."*** I now understand what that means.

The choice is yours. Do you want to enjoy life and have it in abundance or are you going to let the thief continue to steal and kill and destroy you?

I choose life and in abundance. Come on, life is waiting for you. Start living on GO.

TWELVE

God's Timing is Everything

More than five years have passed since I began this book. The first eleven chapters were easy because I was mostly typing out my life as recorded in my journals—this only took a few months. Then the manuscript had to be edited. After changes were made I entered a publishing company contest. My book didn't win. The publishing company offered their services for editing, printing and publishing but that really wasn't what I felt to do at the time.

Someone suggested I print several copies of the manuscript and ask friends and associates to read through and provide suggestions and honest opinions. I asked a relative, a pastor with an editing background, a friend in the broadcasting field and a pastor's wife with editing experience. A total of four people from different walks of life and age brackets read through and gave suggestions.

Then the book sat dormant. I didn't sit dormant but the book wasn't a priority. I felt somehow the book wasn't completed. So I put the draft and the four edited copies in a file.

Until now!

I set my laptop on the island in our kitchen with the four edited copies. As I flipped through page by page, I appreciated the insights provided and made changes where changes needed to be made.

The next step was to reread the book. I made minor adjustments as I went through each page and chapter. Then I came to chapter ten, the chapter about the Phoenix Rising Center. I knew my book wasn't complete—I had to write another chapter about the center.

First I had to go back into my journals and find what I had written about the dream and the vision for the Phoenix Rising Center. I needed to refresh my memory about the whole dream and not just what I shared in chapter ten. Below is exactly what I wrote, about the Phoenix Rising Center.

- 100 acres
- country setting
- large multi-level building (main complex)
- roadway in, trees planted on sides
- large parking lot
- auditorium, 2000 capacity minimum, raised seating
- worship music sound ability
- all rooms in center will have windows
- center with natural healing, Christian
- with counselling
- prayer center/worship/service
- nutrition
- inner healing
- pastors
- iridology
- cancer machines
- baths for mineral salts

- alkaline water
- retreat for both healing, physical and emotional
- covered with prayer
- covered with intercession
- pond with benches
- walking trails
- waterfalls
- Phoenix Rising Center
- iridologists/nutritionists
- teaching center for counsellors
- iridologists
- therapists, live blood
- we all work together
- training center to learn new life skills, die of old, be reborn

I realize there are some duplications but I wanted to write it as written in my journal.

Journaling is so important. I never would have remembered the details and the way God has directed my life since writing chapter ten. The only way to remember little details that somehow become critical later is to journal them as they happen.

As well, you the reader have to realize I put the draft of this book away and went on with life. A lot of living went on between writing the first eleven chapters and writing this chapter.

Our daughter married in August of 2009. The reception took place in our backyard. That summer it rained what seemed like every weekend except, thankfully, the weekend she got married. As you can imagine, spring and summer were extremely busy with all the preparations and garden work. We planted red flowers everywhere to match her colour scheme. I know I said her colour scheme and not their colour scheme but do you really think her fiancé cared about the colour of the flowers we planted?

After the wedding I started thinking about professional development to enhance my skills as a natural health care practitioner. I was leaning towards upgrading in nutrition. At that point, homeopathic medicine wasn't even on my radar. Homeopathic medicine is very specific in symptomatology and every homeopathic medicine matches a certain mental/emotional picture—far too detailed for my liking.

Then one day while I was cleaning out the basement I came across a plastic tote full of books mostly about homeopathic medicine. During prayer at city hall a gentleman who attended periodically, brought me several boxes of books. He was moving out west and didn't want to throw out these books. He thought I would benefit from them. When he gave them to me I skimmed through a few, regarded them as rather complex, and packed them away in this tote.

When I rediscovered the tote, I pulled out book after book and began reading. The examples intrigued me. The books repeatedly described the mental/emotional conditions of my patients, the people who came to me for help. If I had known these things I could have helped my patients more than with just iridology and nutrition. Beyond any doubt many dis-eases are created by the mental/emotional state of a person. What they think about and how they routinely react affects their health and wellness. That is fact.

I felt induced to look further. Homeopathic medicine had my attention.

A quick search on the internet brought me to an introduction to homeopathic medicine at the College of Homeopathic Medicine in

Toronto. I signed up for an online course—no driving back and forth to Toronto for me. I did however have to write my exam in Toronto. Unbeknownst to me this introduction to homeopathic medicine was part of a three-year degree program. By the time I found that out, I was hooked.

As I waited to hear my exam results I explored the idea of taking the three-year degree program which also included a degree in medical health sciences. What was I thinking? Logic said no. I was fifty years old. Toronto seemed a million miles away. I didn't have the money to pay for tuition. I should be saving not spending thousands of dollars as I still had to work to help with the monthly finances of our home. This was impossible. But, somehow after three years, 100,000 kilometres, many grey hairs, many extra pounds added to my figure and five new grandchildren, I graduated. The last semester of my third year I didn't think I would survive but I did.

This week as I type out this chapter I submitted my competencies for full regulation under the College of Homeopaths of Ontario. Homeopathic medicine will soon be regulated under the Regulated Health Professionals Act. You may recall my vision for the clinic involved qualified, certified and accredited natural practitioners. At the time I started the book I was certified as an iridologist but that is not recognized in Ontario. On the other hand, homeopathic medicine is not only recognized but is listed under the Regulated Health Professionals Act. In fact, homeopathic medicine was the first regulated medicine in Ontario—regulated before allopathic medicine or what is called pharmaceutical medicine. Homeopathic medicine was deregulated in the 1970's only to be reregulated in 2007. (I won't get sidetracked here with the political decisions behind this regulation, deregulation and reregulation.)

Do you see how God orchestrated my path? By the way, some of the books in that tote carry valuable information from classic homeopaths and are no longer in print.

As mentioned, the Phoenix Rising Center will maintain a philosophy of working together with medical doctors in a complementary approach. When I first envisioned this, medical doctors were extremely limited regarding any and all complementary approaches to their work. Prior to November of 2011 before the policy was reviewed and updated, the College of Physicians and Surgeons of Ontario policy didn't embrace complementary/alternative medicine readily.

As of November 2011, the policy statement #3-11 states under Introduction, "Patients have the right to make health care decisions that accord with their own values, wishes and preferences. This includes decisions to pursue complementary/alternative medicine either as an adjunct to conventional medicine, or instead of conventional medicine."

Further under 1) Clinical Competency: Knowledge, Skill and Judgement, "Physicians must always act within the limits of their knowledge, skill and judgement and never provide care that is beyond the scope of their clinical competency....

"Where patients seek care that is beyond the physician's clinical competence, physicians must clearly indicate that they are unable to provide the care. Where physicians are unable to provide care directly, they are encouraged to refer the patient to another physician or health-care provider where doing so is in the best interests of the patient, or will support the patient's informed decision making."

In short, if a patient asks a physician to provide complementary care, and they cannot, they can or should refer the patient to a qualified health care provider under the Regulated Health Professionals Act. The Lord knew I needed to be qualified.

Beyond that I have a letter written by the Director for the Health Force Ontario, Ministry of Health and Long-Term Care stating, "The ministry has taken steps to support inter-professional collaboration among health colleges and regulated health professionals. You may be interested to know that HealthForceOntario, the province's health human resources strategy, has identified inter-professional care as an important factor in meeting its objective of ensuring that Ontarians have access to the right number and mix of qualified health care providers."

Now the College of Physicians and Surgeons of Ontario and HealthForceOntario under the Ministry of Health and Long-Term Care are both saying complementary care is the right of each patient.

So what is all the fuss about? Why is it so difficult for this inter-professional care to take place? I can only speak from my professional experience with my patients and drugless cancer care, most physicians don't believe in homeopathic medicine. Yet, homeopathic medicine research has been accepted and written about in oncology journals. In fact one of these studies stated that the four homeopathic medicines used in their study worked as well as Taxol but without the side effects.[1] These aren't new homeopathic medicines but medicines used before pharmaceutical medicine was invented. The homeopathic medicine Ruta has been scientifically proven to cure brain tumours with no side effects. Check out *Ruta 6 ch* on the internet. A report in the US National Library of Medicine National Institutes of Health[2] shows that homeopathic medicine can

[1] http://www.the-cma.org.uk/Articles/Homeopathic-Remedies-Work-To-Kill-Breast-Cancer-Cells-4454/, International Journal of Oncology
[2] http://www.ncbi.nlm.nih.gov/pubmed/18575720

cure lung cancer. Five years ago I couldn't know this and I didn't have the invaluable clinical experience I gained working with patients over the last two years. I've watched patients who have had chemotherapy, radiation, and/or stem cell transplants only to have their cancer return. I've seen the success these same patients gain with homeopathic medicine. As well, I've seen patients who chose not to have chemotherapy or radiation become symptom free using natural protocols. I have the MRI's, ultrasounds and lab work to prove it.

Homeopathic medicine works because it deals with the whole person—physical, mental and emotional. The critical key to success involves pinpointing the issues that helped create the dis-ease in the body. I have seen people who have tried almost everything with little or no success then move on to obtain amazing results with homeopathic medicine. The positive results cannot be denied.

Holistic health care is about the whole body. In my studied opinion based on clinical experience the mental/emotional picture is ninety-five per cent of the whole. The physical symptoms are really just the body saying help. Fears, emotions, worry, stress, anxiety and other emotions play a bigger part than most people realize.

In my journal, I wrote the Phoenix Rising Center needed to accommodate an inner healing, retreat center for physical and emotional healing. Homeopathic medicine and prayer will cover those aspects.

As a homeopath I must follow rules and regulations about what I can and cannot do, and a homeopath is allowed to pray with clients as an added service. My being allowed to pray with people and to work together with physicians would not have been possible five years ago, but today and moving forward it is possible.

In my journal the list of points about the Phoenix Rising Centre also included live blood analysis. At the time I had little or no concept of the importance of this, but after my training I realize the significance of regular live blood analysis.

A year ago I was *prompted* to purchase a microscope. I practised on myself and family members. Then I took a course on live blood analysis. This proved critical and invaluable for my drugless cancer care patients. You may think this co-incidental, but I know God is directing my path.

Is the Phoenix Rising Center any closer to being built? Yes. I see it in my prayers, hopes and dreams. I believe it more than ever. We are five years closer to completion. I see the big picture. I see the center completed. That is my gift. When people read this book, those with the necessary skills to make the vision happen will come on board. We will work together by God's grace and watch His mighty hand clear the way. I believe it is closer then we know.

A year or so ago a patient of mine phoned and asked me to look at his piece of land, valued at about $400,000. He was considering donating it for the Phoenix Rising Center. He asked that I view the property and pray about it.

You might think after all these years I would jump at this opportunity. I drove to the property, walked around and prayed. It didn't feel right. Even though the land was offered I still needed confirmation that it was the right property. Confirmation didn't come.

I am confident the right property and the funding are on the way.

Not long ago while in prayer I felt the Holy Spirit direct me to look at the mission statement of St. Joseph's hospital in Hamilton Ontario. It identifies the hospital as "a Catholic hospital, owned and operated by the St. Joseph's Health System and committed to carrying out the healing mission of Jesus Christ." The mission statement goes on to say, "We are dedicated to providing compassionate, sensitive care to our patients and their families and to achieving excellence in health care through our on-going commitment to education and research."

Their Vision: "On behalf of those we are privileged to serve, we will deliver an integrated high quality care experience, pursue and share knowledge, and respect our rich diversity, always remaining faithful to our Roman Catholic values and traditions."

The Phoenix Rising Center could very easily adopt this mission statement. My point being, St. Joseph's Hospital is incorporated and has charitable status as a non-profit, as does Phoenix Rising Center. People give donations to St. Joseph's Hospital and they can also give to the Phoenix Rising Center and receive a similar charitable tax receipt. St. Joseph's hospital gets funding from the provincial government as do other hospitals in Hamilton. If they receive funding why can't the Phoenix Rising Center?

The St. Joseph's hospital began when the sister of St. Joseph's saw a need in the community. They acted on the need, built and looked after the administration of the hospital. This is what the Phoenix Rising Center purposes to do—meet a need in the community today. HealthForceOntario recognized the need of inter-professional collaboration among regulated health practitioners; the Ministry of Health and Long-Term Care recognized the need to reregulate homeopathic medicine; and the Phoenix Rising Center will be built to fulfill the need for Drugless Cancer Care.

I follow some of the protocols of Eli G. Jones, M.D. from his book, *CANCER, Its Causes, Symptoms and Treatment*. This book presents the results obtained during more than forty years experience in the medical treatment of this disease. In his book he describes the vision of a facility similar to the Phoenix Rising Center. By the way, the four successful homeopathic medicines that were used in research at the M.D. Anderson Cancer Center in Houston, Texas are among those used by Eli G, Jones M.D. in the late 1800's and early 1900's to cure breast cancer as stated in his book.

In chapter ten I mentioned a dream and some of the dream I was not ready or willing to share. That still stands, but I will share this. At the end of the dream or interpretation of the dream I have written, "BE BOLD." When I reread those words I remember I had that prayed over me, not once but twice at two different conferences in two different countries concerning two different sets of circumstances.

I needed a reminder to BE BOLD. Perhaps it's time to BE BOLDER!

I dedicate this book to my eight grandchildren; Travis, Owen, Teegan, Cailyn, Ryder, Kason, Ryleigh and River. My prayer is that you have a deep personal relationship with Jesus and that you trust Him with all your hopes and dreams. Always go for what you believe in your heart and never, ever give up.

Through all the crazy in my life you have always been there. I thank you for your love, support and words of caution. I wouldn't have been able to do what I have accomplished without you Randy my loving husband.

With all my love Diane

To book Diane Elms to speak at your next event,
contact
founder@phoenixrisingcenter.ca
or
founder@phoenixrisingcenter.com
or
905-768-0848